# After Stroke

# After Stroke

The Complete, Step-by-step Blueprint for Getting Better

David M. Hinds

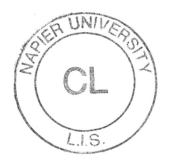

Thorsons

Thorsons
An Imprint of HarperCollins*Publishers*
77–85 Fulham Palace Road
Hammersmith, London W6 8JB

The Thorsons website address is www.thorsons.com

Published by Thorsons 2000

10 9 8 7 6 5 4 3 2 1

© David M. Hinds 2000

David M. Hinds asserts the moral right to
be identified as the author of this work

A catalogue record for this book is available
from the British Library

ISBN 0 7225 3885 5

Printed and bound by
Caledonian International Book Manufacturing Ltd, Glasgow

To my daughters, Johanna and Danielle,
and my long lost son, Jason.

**Important Note**

This book is not intended to be a substitute for medical advice or treatment. Any person with a condition requiring medical attention should consult a qualified medical practitioner.

# Contents

## part three • Denial

## part four • Anger

## part five • Guilt

## part seven • Depression

## part eight • Adjustment

## part nine • Wellbeing

## Sources of help and support

# Acknowledgements

Grateful acknowledgement is given for permission to reproduce illustrations and instructions from The Stroke Association's *Get Moving* booklet by Sarah Tyson, Ann Ashburn and Jacqueline Jackson, with line drawings by Juliet Baker. I should also like to thank The Stroke Association for their help and support during the writing of this book.

I am indebted to Professor Sir Peter Morris and his team at the John Radcliffe Hospital, Oxford, for their care when my carotid artery was completely blocked and destroyed by stroke. My gratitude, also, to Professor Morris for agreeing to write a foreword to this book.

Finally, I would like to thank Derek Campbell at the Polperro Bookshop and Café who patiently guided and coaxed me into producing my best, and the magnificent staff of the Cornwall Reference Library in Truro for their unfailing enthusiasm in researching and providing information.

# Foreword

I first met David Hinds early in August 1995 following his major stroke, which had been preceded, by a minor stroke a day or two before. He was referred for consideration of surgical reconstruction of the blood flow to his brain.

As you might imagine, over that few months I saw a great deal of David. He was a relatively young man who had had a very busy lifestyle and a very successful career, but who was slowly realising that his career, and even perhaps his life, was in ruins. Needless to say, he was extremely angry about this and early on unavoidably showed this in his relationships with his carers. However, what was fascinating was that over those early weeks as all the problems that he had began to sink in (which are so well described in this book), he began to consider how he could adjust his life to cope with his disability, and what he could do to minimise his disabilities. In this remarkable book he describes his reaction to the stroke and how he managed to cope with all the problems associated with a major stroke.

He has now made an excellent recovery and has established a new lifestyle for himself. This book is not only a record of his own experiences of coping with a stroke, but also a distillation of a vast amount of reading and discussion on the subject. Furthermore, it is expressed in a way that will make it invaluable not only for people who have had a stroke, but also for their carers.

Peter J. Morris, FRCS, FRS
Nuffield Professor of Surgery
University of Oxford

# Introduction

Every year in Britain, 100,000 people have a stroke. In the United States, 400,000 suffer. The physical and emotional impact of the illness on patients and carers is enormous. Seventy per cent of stroke patients survive but many are severely brain-damaged and disabled. The purpose of this book is to inspire and motivate the 10.7 million annual survivors of stroke worldwide into making the best possible recovery available to them. For the vast majority of patients with the capacity to recover, it is possible to reclaim their health and lifestyle providing they possess the will to get well and a genuine willingness to struggle. This patient-centred book will help.

The nine parts of this book coincide with the principal psychological effects of actually experiencing a stroke. The mental response to suffering a stroke is fundamentally a grief reaction. The patient is mourning the loss of faculties, lifestyle and status.

Grief, a natural human reaction to loss, is a process of adaptation and passes through a number of recognizable stages, regardless of whether the loss is a loved one, amputation or paralysis. These stages include *alarm, shock, denial, anger, guilt, acceptance* and *adjustment.* The majority of stroke patients also go through a period of *depression.* Sadly, at present, too few patients and carers reach the final stage of *wellbeing. After Stroke* will steer readers towards this positive outcome.

I have personally made a 100-per-cent recovery from two major strokes and a subclavian bypass operation. I hope that you will find this book helpful and easy to read. My aim is to reveal the inside story, the know-how, the essential steps to recovery, with humour, frankness and authority. I want to reach out to a stroke victim's feelings of frustration, distress and depression from the depth of personal experience, moving patients and carers resolutely onward. The book is focused on total recovery from stroke, nothing less.

# PART ONE
# alarm

# 1 : You are never too old to recover from stroke

*Great emergencies and crises show us how much greater our vital resources are than we had supposed.*

William James 1842–1910

You are never too old to recover from stroke: not everyone can make a complete recovery, but most of us, over time, can manage a major improvement in our condition. The keys to a quality life after stroke are support, guidance, rehabilitation and, most important of all, the will to get well. For those of us who are alone in the world, the will to get well can be the deciding factor.

The first 10 days after stroke are the most cruel. After that, with adequate aftercare and the right attitude of mind, things can get progressively better. Make no mistake, recovering from stroke is never easy. For some it will prove to be the toughest challenge of their lives. But for the chance to win back our health, with all the rewards, opportunities, and treats that will accompany success, are we not willing to do *whatever it takes* to get well?

Just for a moment, let us suppose that the forthcoming struggle to recover our health will be an adventure, not an impossibility. In order to understand how and why, at almost any age, we have a phenomenal ability to recover from stroke, allow me to give you an insight to what is happening inside your brain. You may be reassured to discover that your brain is quite capable of navigating around the stroke-damaged areas of itself in much the same way that you might take a detour if your usual route home was blocked by an accident. Your brain has spare capacity for emergencies such as this.

### THE BOTTOM LINE

Commit to the best possible recovery *you* can manage.

Damage by stroke occurs only in the brain. Nothing at all has happened to the muscles. They malfunction on one side of the body after stroke because they are not getting the usual messages for movement from the brain. With time, physiotherapy and perseverance, the stroke patient who survives the initial trauma can often recover lost or impaired faculties as the brain finds alternative pathways around the damaged areas.

I know only too well from my own experiences of recovering from two strokes that you must be feeling frustrated and frightened right now. A stroke defies definition in so many ways. No two strokes are the same. Suddenly, unexpectedly, your whole life implodes. The saddest thing about stroke is that your nearest and dearest can help you but they can't enter into the struggle. No one but you can win.

Despite your misfortune, if you can somehow summon the will to read on, this book will hold your good hand and guide you every step of the way through the marvels of your own recovery. The essential first step is to commit your heart and soul to recovery, the best possible recovery that *you* can manage.

# 2: Let's cut off the blood supply to the brain

*If anything can go wrong,
it will, and at the most
inopportune time.*
Murphy's Law

The majority of readers of this book will be stroke patients, their carers, family and friends. If you are reading this book as a stroke patient then you are indeed doing well. **You *are* a survivor!** The road to recovery and wellbeing after stroke may well be a difficult one, but I can assure you with absolute sincerity that it is worthwhile to struggle. Following almost total recovery from my second major stroke three years ago, I am happier now than ever before.

---

A BASIC UNDERSTANDING OF WHAT HAS HAPPENED TO THE PATIENT WILL BENEFIT US ALL.
**Let's cut off the blood supply to the brain and simulate a stroke!**

---

When the blood supply to the brain is interrupted, a complex series of metabolic processes takes place and calcium poisons a cluster of brain cells, accelerating their demise. At first those cells under siege from blood starvation remain alive but cease to function properly. Within four to eight minutes, irreversible damage results and cells in the affected part of the brain inevitably expire.

At the fundamental cell level, a human brain might be compared to a computer. After all, computers are essentially a series of tiny switches that can be

**THE BOTTOM LINE**

Hang on to your sense of humour.
You'll be needing it.

programmed for either 'on' or 'off', depending on the task to be performed. Likewise, our brain cells (or neurons to be precise) either 'fire', discharging an electrochemical signal for some kind of action to take place (the movement of a finger, for instance), or 'do not fire', if no change is required. It is this interruption to the orderly flow of brain signals caused by defunct and damaged cells that plays havoc with one side of the body after stroke.

Unlike the cells in the tissues of our skin or liver which can usually reproduce those lost through damage, once an adult loses a brain cell it is gone forever. Fortunately, most of us have a few billion of them. To get around the effects of brain damage caused by stroke, patients must try to retrain undamaged brain cells to take on new roles, such as controlling their muscle movements to facilitate walking. This can be easier than it sounds because the connections between brain cells become more sensitive close to the area that has been destroyed. Also, swelling around the grey matter in the skull will subside. When this happens, the less damaged brain cells regain their function and your recovery accelerates.

It will take time, determination and, in many cases, the intervention of a highly-skilled physiotherapist before other brain cells mirror the performance of cells consumed by stroke and mobility can be restored. For the benefit of every patient with the capacity to recover from stroke and, so important, the will, the step-by-step road to recovery is here within the pages of *After Stroke*.

# 3: CAUTION: brain attack

*Even if the prospects seem bad,*
*you have to carry on.*

General Eisenhower 1890–1969

When the blood supply to our brain is interrupted, a 'brain attack' occurs. Usually this happens because a blood clot blocks an artery, but it can be caused by bleeding directly into the brain. The experience is sometimes fatal, often devastating, but never painful. Surprisingly, our human brains are not supplied with pain receptors!

The medical term for a brain attack is stroke and most people are conscious when it happens. Loss of consciousness may result in a minority of serious cases and many strokes take place when the individual is sleeping. The majority of patients, although dazed and confused, can vividly recall the onset of stroke. Even now, three years after the event, I can remember every last detail ...

It had been a glorious summer's day in August. Enjoying the solitude and tranquillity of my own company, I had taken a leisurely stroll in the woods before stopping for lunch. Just after 10 o'clock that evening, as I sat alone in my study at home preparing my workload for Monday, I reached forward for a glass of water on my desk, spilling it all over my paperwork.

Not entirely at once, but gradually, in terrifying waves of panic, I became aware that part of one side of my body was paralysed. I could barely move or control my quivering lips, from which saliva was escaping. The two sides of my mouth were shuddering involuntarily, but not in harmony: one side more sluggish than the other. I couldn't understand why, according to the clock facing me, half-an-hour seemed to have elapsed in the time it had taken me to

**THE BOTTOM LINE**

## Seek urgent medical advice.

mop up the spillage with my handkerchief.

The right half of my body felt numb and heavy and my face didn't seem to fit any more. It occurred to me that maybe I should call a doctor, but then, I wondered, if I went to bed, perhaps I would be all right in the morning.

When, as if in a dream, or rather a nightmare, I probed myself disbelievingly with a finger that worked, I discovered that one corner of my mouth was an inch higher than the other. I cursed and swore, or rather I tried to, but all that would come out was gibberish! It dawned on me that I was living a nightmare, not dreaming it.

# 4: EMERGENCY: stroke in progress

*Happiness alone is beneficial for the body, but it is grief that develops the powers of the mind.*

Marcel Proust 1871–1922

Don't believe the cynics who say nothing can be done about stroke. There is much that can be achieved both to rehabilitate the patient and to dramatically reduce the risk of another stroke. The first priority is to get immediate medical assessment. The vast majority of stroke patients will need to be admitted to hospital.

The right side of the brain controls the left side of the body. This means that a stroke affecting the right side of the brain will affect the left side of the body and vice versa. When someone suffers a stroke, what we see are the outward signs of brain damage that occurs when the blood supply to the brain has been cut off. There are three immediate features:

**THE BOTTOM LINE**

## Don't hesitate: call a doctor.

- STROKE IS SUDDEN. The physical effects of stroke become instantaneously obvious and can include weakness or paralysis of the arm and leg on one side of the body and twisting of the face. In some cases there are other effects such as loss of balance, disturbance of vision or speech and difficulty in swallowing.
- STROKE INVOLVES THE BRAIN. Although what we are seeing is bodily malfunctioning, the damage nevertheless is in the brain. There is no actual injury to the muscles. They are affected only as a consequence of brain damage.
- STROKE INFLUENCES OUR MENTAL STATE. To be confused and tired is usual following a stroke.

---

**You need to know**

- Your doctor cannot be expected to make an accurate prediction of how long it will take you to recover. Some patients find that their condition improves considerably in the early weeks following their stroke.
- You should not be discouraged if your recovery seems to be slow. It may take a very long time indeed (perhaps as much as three years) and consistent effort on your part to complete the best possible recovery that *you* can manage.

---

## *Rapid recovery tips*

1) Try to relax, keep calm and stop worrying. I know, in your present predicament, this will be difficult advice to follow, but it is by far the most important single tip I can give you. If you worry you will succeed only in slowing down your ability to get well.

2) Simplify your life or get others to do it for you. Your priorities have changed. For the time being all that matters is getting well. Let *nothing* interfere with that one overriding priority.

3) Get plenty of rest. You will feel tired and easily exhausted in the months following stroke.

# 5: Why me?

*Our safety and our peril*
*lie in ourselves.*

Epictetus AD 50–120

Do any of the following known causes of stroke apply to you, the stroke patient? Or to your patient if you are the generous-hearted one caring for another? In order to get well and stay that way, we are going to have to ask ourselves some pretty searching questions about our own personal preferences and habits and the way we conduct our lives. To be effective in convalescence, it may be necessary to make some changes to our lifestyle and even perhaps to our approach and attitude to life itself.

The list of risk factors for stroke on page 10 is likely to be the uncomfortable moment of truth for many people, as indeed it was for me when I first saw it. Providing we are willing to be completely open and candid with ourselves, it can also be the start of a new, healthier chapter in our lives. The beginning of a new beginning.

All you need to do now is simply underline the words on the following page that you think may apply to you. Or your carer can do it for you. Don't apportion blame to yourself or anyone else.

**THE BOTTOM LINE**

## Is this me? Yes it is, but I'll be back!

## Could this be you? Risk factors for stroke

- HIGH BLOOD PRESSURE. This is the most important risk factor of all. If your pressure is too high (consistently more than 135/85) it weakens and damages arteries, making them more likely to burst. Have your blood pressure checked regularly.
- NARROW ARTERIES. Blood clots can form and lodge in arteries that are clogged and hardened with deposits of fat.
- SMOKING. The more you smoke, the higher the risk. Cessation is the only answer.
- ALCOHOL. Regular heavy drinking and bingeing raises blood pressure.
- HEART DISEASE. Patients with a history of heart problems including heart attacks, abnormal heart valves and irregularity of heartbeat are more vulnerable to clots.
- PREVIOUS STROKE OR MINI-STROKE. Did you take steps to reduce your risk?
- PHYSICAL INACTIVITY. Lack of exercise doubles your risk of stroke.
- UNHEALTHY DIET. Saturated fats, too much salt, fat on meat, oven-ready and processed foods can cause arterial problems. A daily intake of fresh fruit and vegetables and a varied diet including cereals and oily fish twice a week is your healthiest option.
- DIABETES accelerates narrowing of the arteries and doubles the risk of stroke.
- ORAL CONTRACEPTIVES raise the risk of stroke only slightly.
- HORMONE REPLACEMENT THERAPY is believed to carry a slight risk of stroke but existing data is not conclusive.
- MIGRAINE IN WOMEN. Young women with a history of migraine are three-and-a-half times more likely to suffer an ischemic stroke according to new research from the Imperial College School of Medicine and the Radcliffe Infirmary.

# 6: Mini-stroke: THE ULTIMATE WARNING

*There is no good in arguing with the inevitable. The only argument available with an east wind is to put on your overcoat.*

James Russell Lowell 1819–91

Mini-strokes – often referred to in medical terms as transient ischemic attacks (TIAs) – last less than 24 hours and do not kill. *They are a warning!* Their significance is that they can be followed by a full-blown stroke.

High blood pressure is the most important risk factor in stroke. The best thing you can do to reduce the risk of stroke is to have your blood pressure checked without delay. Next, you should look closely at your lifestyle and diet. Changing the habits of a lifetime is never easy but it can be a walk in the park compared to the trauma of stroke.

Many strokes are preceded by brief episodes where the individual experiences a sudden disturbance of speech or vision or weakness on one side of the body. Typically there may be a momentary loss of vision, not unlike the effect of a veil descending in front of the eye or a sphere of sparkling diamonds. Speech can sound slurred to others but not necessarily to the person affected. One arm or leg and possibly one side of the mouth or face may feel weak, paralysed, heavy or slightly prickly.

What often happens is that the symptoms disappear, the patient heaves a sigh of relief, life continues as usual and your doctor, lacking in psychic powers, is none the wiser. What should happen is that you report the occurrence to

## THE BOTTOM LINE

See your doctor and have your blood pressure checked.

your GP. You won't know if you are at risk unless you have your blood pressure checked regularly. A word of warning. Ask your GP to check the pressure of each arm in case you are one of those rare unfortunates (like me) with high blood pressure on one side and lower blood pressure on the other. I have a bitter memory of being congratulated by a nurse for having almost normal blood pressure one week and being hospitalized by stroke the next. Needless to say, I held out the wrong arm!

Migraine, particularly in young women, increases the risk of an ischemic stroke. This occurs when blocked blood vessels constrict blood flow to the brain. Migraine is common the world over and is six times more prevalent than diabetes. Three times as many women as men are migraine sufferers and most experience their first attack between their early teens and the age of 40. Those at risk should contact their GP and the *Managing Migraine Service* which is designed specifically for sufferers.

Take action now to reduce the risk of further strokes. Be aware that risk factors don't just add up, they multiply! For instance, someone with high blood pressure has up to seven times the risk of stroke, whereas an average cigarette smoker with correspondingly high blood pressure is doubly (14 times) at risk. But a smoker with very high blood pressure (hypertension) has **28 times the risk of stroke!!!**

# 7: Stroke in the younger generation

> *The individual who is able to perceive a glimmer of possibility in a situation that seems, at first glance, full of insurmountable obstacles, is the one who is most likely to reap the greatest benefits.*
>
> John Paul Getty 1892–1976

The bottom line, below, to a youngster who has suddenly and inexplicably met with misfortune, might seem a bit rich, if not downright insensitive. Before finding success in my 30s, and greater success in my 40s, I made a complete hash of my teens. After one particularly spectacular escapade that ended in disaster and hospitalization for many months, someone for whom I had the greatest respect said to me: 'One day you'll look back at this time in your life and laugh.' I thought he was heartless, but in fact he was right.

Look once again at the bottom line below. You cannot be expected to believe in the wisdom of those words right now – *you're hurting so much* – but in time you can be in a position to benefit.

Throughout the ages, people of all generations have been suffering strokes. Around 400 BC the Greek physician, Hippocrates, commonly regarded as the father of medicine, wrote that many Greeks suffered apoplexy. This is a sudden, extraordinary attack on the senses, known today as a 'brain attack' or stroke.

Without warning, stroke causes instant disability from which most of us, if

**THE BOTTOM LINE**

## This setback can and will strengthen your character.

we have the will to do so, can eventually recover mobility (the younger you are, the greater your chances of making a complete recovery).

Stroke can also be soul-shattering, and that is often harder to come to terms with than the physical damage. Getting back to normal will involve a traumatic journey from here to a place where life can be meaningful and worthwhile once again. Of necessity, this will mean an unplanned expedition, a deviation from the expected course of our young lives, in order to turn misfortune around and triumph over adversity. This is the part that can mould and strengthen character and eventually pay a handsome bonus. No matter how serious or superficial your stroke, in addition to the capacity to recover, you will need to embrace The Three 'P's in order to derive ultimate benefit from *the bottom line.*

## The Three 'P's

PATIENCE
POSITIVE ATTITUDE
PERSEVERANCE

Recovery from stroke can be slow. Inactive or malfunctioning limbs cannot be 'switched on'. Mobility is regained gradually. The leg usually recovers before the arm and the arm before the hand. Doctors are initially reluctant to predict the extent of eventual recovery. This is because it is not possible to make an accurate forecast until two or three weeks after stroke. In younger patients, if the process of rehabilitation takes a long time, it may be several years before complete recovery or the final degree of independence is achieved. Much depends on the attitude and motivation of the patient.

# 8: Stroke in retirement

*Although the world is full of suffering, it is full also of the overcoming of it.*

Helen Keller 1880–1968

On the one hand, it is usually harder for older people to learn new ways of doing things, to adapt to change, and to recover from stroke. On the other, the older generation are a wily lot: they have known tough times before! Unlike younger patients, they have recourse to a lifetime of wisdom and experience. They can draw upon this valuable reserve to help them towards recovery, even stealing a march on their younger counterparts.

The fact is that you are never too old to recover from stroke. What you need now to help you get better is some good, old-fashioned, down-to-earth know-how. You must always follow your doctor's advice and, if in doubt, ask for guidance. Your doctor is the practitioner who has access to your full medical history and knows what is best for you in your particular case. The combination of sound medical advice and the practical guidance given in these pages will tip the scales firmly in your favour.

Consider the cases of two grand senior citizens and a Hollywood film star, all of whom have recovered from stroke:

**Sir John Harvey-Jones** was the high-profile chairman of the world-ranking British pharmaceutical company, ICI, until his retirement in 1990. Thanks to a very successful television series which featured his troubleshooting skills, he became a household name. In 1994 he suffered two strokes and has since recovered remarkably well. Now 74, he had this to say in *Stroke News*, published by The Stroke Association:

**THE BOTTOM LINE**

## Be gentle with yourself and others.

A stroke does mean that you have lost a little of your brain power so you are not quite the person you used to be. But there is a very big difference between that and being useless. I'm still doing all the same things as I was before the strokes, but at a slower pace.

**Admiral Sir Richard Thomas.** Due to the televising of the proceedings of the British Houses of Parliament, the ceremonial office of Black Rod in the House of Lords is familiar to a large public. In 1993, the holder of the post, Admiral Sir Richard Thomas, had a severe stroke at the age of 61. The stroke left him paralysed on one side and slightly affected his speech. He spent five-and-a-half months in hospital and returned to his post two weeks later. He had this to say in *Stroke News*:

> My job required me to be on ceremonial parade every day so it was very important to get my walking passable if not perfect. That gave me the motivation I needed during rehabilitation. A problem with stroke is that nobody seems to have the aim of getting you as near as possible back to normal. It is still too readily accepted that the disabilities you have will be with you for the rest of your life. **I believe that attitude should be challenged.**

When **Patricia Neal,** the film star, was hit by a series of strokes and came home to England after being in hospital in California, she could not read or write or handle numbers. At Heathrow Airport she was met by about 50 reporters and cameramen and was compelled to hold a sort of press conference. In a foreword to the book *A Stroke in the Family* by Valerie Eaton Griffith (published by The Stroke Association), Pat's husband, Roald Dahl, recalled that it was a crazy affair because Pat was not only crippled but also unable to answer questions except in monosyllables. When Roald announced that one day his wife would act again, the assembled media became silent. The reporters stared. The reaction was as if he had announced that the woman was about to sprout wings and fly to the moon.

Three years later, Pat walked onto the stage of the Waldorf-Astoria in New York and the place exploded. To the audience, she was back from the dead and they were cheering not only the woman herself but also the comforting thought that it is possible for anyone, given a lot of guts and a bit of luck, to overcome gigantic misfortunes and terrible illness. She had done it. And that meant others could do the same.

# 9: Tips for coping in a crisis

*Now we can look the East End in the face.*
Queen Elizabeth the Queen Mother surveying the damage caused to Buckingham Palace by a bomb during the Blitz. 1900–

One of the greatest causes of stress in life is change, and a stroke in the family inevitably means *change!* Laughable as it may seem for both patient and carer, your greatest asset in the difficult days ahead will be a sense of humour. If, despite misfortune, you can endeavour to see the funny side of efforts that misfire, this will dramatically ease the tension and help you both to pull through.

For the patient, the first rule of survival when tragedy strikes is to keep calm and simplify life. All that matters now is getting well and staying cool. Delegate, or get others to delegate for you, *anything* that is not directly connected with getting better or surviving this crisis.

It is also essential for the wellbeing of the carer to have proper breaks away from the responsibility of looking after the patient. If you think you cannot afford to take time out for yourself then that is probably a sure sign that you need a break. Ask friends to cover for you.

**THE BOTTOM LINE**

Stay calm, don't panic, concentrate on priorities.

- Carer beware of these killer phrases: 'I'm fine', 'Don't bother', 'I can manage', 'I'm all right'…
- Ask yourself: Are you making life unnecessarily difficult for yourself?
- Would you like some help? The next time someone offers, try saying: 'Yes please'.

To the non-professional carer, thrown in at the deep end by fate, problems can at first seem overwhelming. There is no need to panic. Problems are much easier to handle if given a name and identity. If something is bothering you, focus all your attention on it and define exactly what the problem is. Write it down and give it a name. Regardless of whether it is an awful problem, or something that others might consider to be comparatively trivial, you are already making great progress. No longer do you have a cloud of anxiety hanging over your head, you have a specific problem on a piece of paper. Now all you need is a solution.

## Problem-solving devices

- When faced with a problem, check that it is indeed *your* problem for *you* to deal with.
- Scan the back pages of this book for sources of help and guidance.
- Is it a *money* problem? If so, find out if you are entitled to financial assistance (in the UK, call The Benefits Enquiry Line).
- Do you need independent help? Consult a professional therapist or counsellor.
- When changes are needed, pick the easiest thing first and *do it*.
- Most important of all, share your worries with a friend whenever possible

# 10: Unloading your worries

*I like a man what takes
his time.*
Mae West 1892–1980

When tragedy strikes, most people, no matter how talented or down-to-earth, haven't got a clue how *not* to worry. I know this for certain from my pre-stroke days as a stress management consultant and counsellor. How to cope effectively in an emergency, without unnecessary worrying, is a skill that can and must be learned in order to accelerate the process of recovery. If you do worry when recuperating from stroke (the temptation and natural tendency is to do just that) you will succeed only in slowing down your improvement.

Of course, it is easy to say stop worrying. But how? Here is a technique which many people have found useful. It's a mind game for everyone.

Just for a moment or two – longer, if you can manage it – imagine your worries listed on one single sheet of paper. When you've reached the bottom of this page, picture yourself placing that sheet of paper, complete with all your worries, under your pillow or on the mantelpiece (or anywhere you choose)…*There*, where you can keep an eye on them if you want to, but where they can no longer drag you down into the doldrums because **they** *are no longer a part of* **you**.

Don't hesitate. Play this simple mind game even if you don't usually indulge in such things. After all, what have you got to lose – your troubles? You can always pick them up later for a Titanic worrying session if you must. Who knows? One day you might forget where you put them. You may even decide that you can do without them. The same is true for carers. Caring and constructive action is positive. Worrying is self-defeating and pointless: **an indulgence you can't afford.**

### THE BOTTOM LINE

# Essential medicine: relax, take it easy, try not to worry.

## Read this sequence and try it

- Briefly remind yourself what your worries are.
- Look around you and select a place to leave your single sheet of worries.
- Lie back and close your eyes.
- Imagine yourself off-loading all your worries to that place then heave a sigh of relief.
- Take a deep breath and exhale slowly. Open your eyes and force yourself to smile.
- You're on the road to recovery. Read *on* with the weight *off* your shoulders.

# PART TWO
# shock

# 1: Getting through the worst: the first 10 days

*Some patients, though conscious that their condition is perilous, recover their health simply through their contentment with the goodness of the physician.*

Hippocrates 460–377 BC

No two strokes are exactly the same, but one thing is the same for all stroke survivors and their loved ones: the first 10 days are the worst. In order to weather the aftermath of stroke and establish a basis on which to recover, four factors must come into play.

The patient must have:
- access to immediate and ongoing medical care
- the expectation of getting better
- the will to recover, even if the going gets tough
- as little to worry about as possible.

When hospitalized by two strokes in 1995, I was lucky in as much that my knowledge of stress management and counselling came to my rescue and significantly aided my recovery. For once in my life I practised what I had been preaching to everyone else for years and cut out the unnecessary clutter from my daily existence. With two simple but supremely difficult to pronounce

**THE BOTTOM LINE**

Simplify your life and **expect** to get better.

instructions (one to my solicitor and the other to an estate agent recommended by a nurse) I relieved myself of all pressure so that I could focus on the one thing that really mattered: **getting well.**

I was living alone at the time of my illness. Other than my health, or rather the lack of it, I had only two problems that were troubling me: my unnecessarily large house with mortgage to match and my stress management consultancy. I sold one and closed the other.

After stroke, patients experience different rates and degrees of improvement. Some patients, even major stroke patients, make an almost complete recovery, while others are left with some impairment. The emotional impact of stroke is much the same as surviving a major accident. Tears, frustration, anger, revulsion, feelings of helplessness and lack of confidence may follow a prolonged period of numbness, shock and disbelief. Fear of further strokes and depression are all-too-frequent visitors to the shell-shocked mind of the patient.

Remember, that after a major life-threatening event of any kind, probably none of us is ever quite the same again. Both patient and carer may have to adjust to a new situation. Although change, any change of lifestyle or routine, is stressful, it can also be surprisingly rewarding and beneficial in time. I tell you this with 100 per cent conviction. After three years of upheaval and uncertainty following my discharge from hospital, I am happier now than ever before.

# 2: The causes of stroke

> *Each player must accept the cards life deals him or her. But once they are in hand, he or she alone must decide how to play the cards ...*
>
> Voltaire 1694–1778

The causes of stroke are most easily understood when categorized as three primary sets of risk factors: those which you can do something about yourself, risks factors that neither you nor your doctor can change, and those which your doctor can effectively help you to reduce.

For every ten people who die from stroke, four might have been saved by having regular blood pressure checks and by following their doctors' advice (including taking medication, if prescribed) to bring their blood pressure down. So many strokes, including second and subsequent strokes, could be avoided if those at risk took immediate steps to reduce their exposure to the main risk factors, listed below.

## Risk factors which you can do something about yourself

- **SMOKING.** The only effective solution is to quit. Smoking causes furring up of the arteries and makes the blood more likely to clot. Smoking doubles your risk of stroke, but the benefits of quitting are immediate: your risk of stroke starts to diminish straight away.
- **LACK OF PHYSICAL EXERCISE.** A lifestyle of physical inactivity is linked to high blood pressure, the cause of many strokes. Regular physical

**THE BOTTOM LINE**

All is not lost: you are still in the game.

activity is good for you but it is most beneficial if you work or play hard enough to get slightly breathless.

- **UNHEALTHY DIET.** Excessive consumption of salt is linked to high blood pressure while fatty foods can cause blood clots to form and lodge in narrowed arteries. A diet rich in fresh fruit and vegetables or Mediterranean-style diet may help protect against stroke.
- **DRINKING TOO MUCH ALCOHOL.** Indulging in 'binge-drinking' is a major risk factor, increasing the risk of stroke five-fold. Regular heavy drinking also increases the risk of stroke, whereas the moderate consumption of alcohol does not.

## Risk factors that neither you nor your doctor can change

- **AGE.** Stroke can affect anyone of any age, but older people are at greater risk.
- **ORIGIN.** Stroke illness is common all over the world, but people of Asian or Afro-Caribbean origin are at higher risk.
- **PARENTAGE.** Descendants of those with a history of stroke are more vulnerable.

## Risk factors your doctor can help you to reduce

- **HIGH BLOOD PRESSURE** and hypertension.
- **MINI-STROKE** (transient ischemic attack), narrowing of the arteries and heart problems.
- **MIGRAINE**, diabetes and oral contraception (the risk factor for some types of oral contraception is minimal).

Don't hesitate to visit your doctor to discuss ways of reducing your risk of stroke. Remember, it is up to you to make the first move. Make an appointment to visit the surgery.

# 3: The effects of stroke

*Chaos often breeds life,*
*when order breeds habit.*
Henry Adams 1838–1918

Until recently, stroke was regarded with despair, with no effective options for treatment. This attitude is being swept aside as new prospects for prevention, acute treatment and rehabilitation come to the fore. There is an emerging trend towards more dynamic stroke management, and this important development is acknowledged in the 1998 Scrip Report: *Pathways to Future Therapy* by Ruth Kirby.

The effects of stroke can vary greatly from one patient to another. Three irreversible factors govern the severity of stroke illness: *how much of the brain is damaged, the particular part of the brain involved and the age of the patient.*

A glance down the table of contents at the front of the book will give you an insight to the diversity of deficits that can be sustained by just one stroke. Fortunately, very few patients have to contend with all of these difficulties at once. Some, against all odds, succeed beyond the wildest expectations of their loved ones to regain almost complete health in a few short months or years. Humbled by the experience of cheating death and disability by a whisker, they are invariably wiser and more humane, like battle-weary war veterans, returning from hell.

Each of the perverse and disagreeable effects of stroke, and how best to overcome their unique challenges, will be explained later in the book. On this page, I seek only to alert readers to the deceptive and tricky nature of the illness and to warn you of the difficulties ahead so that you will not be floored by the trying, sometimes cruel, and frequently outrageous nature of the illness.

**THE BOTTOM LINE**

## Beyond chaos you may find contentment.

After stroke, almost everyone, to some extent, suffers from tiredness and a lack of energy. The problem is mainly confined to the initial period of recovery but exhaustion can be a persistent problem which affects the patient's day-to-day existence for months or years to come. Many patients complain of physical, emotional and mental tiredness after stroke and it is possible to experience all three together. I myself can testify to the mayhem caused by that recovery-limiting trio, but carer *beware*! There is a natural disinclination to put strain on the patient and a feeling that constant rest is necessary. This can have precisely the wrong effect. It goes without saying that stroke patients must be allowed their privacy, their dignity and frequent periods of rest, but for their own good they may have to be treated with firmness. Total recovery is more likely to be achieved if effort is exerted by the patient **sooner rather than later**.

# 4: Will I recover, and when?

*Healing is a matter of time,*
*but it is sometimes also a*
*matter of opportunity.*
Hippocrates 460–377 BC

Whether the patient recovers, and when, depends, in my experience, as much on faith, laughter and support, as on the healing abilities of the body or physician. If the patient's mindset is attuned to recovery, the very best that can be achieved, a lifeline to recovery is already established. Not for this patient, when the time comes to get back behind the wheel of a car, a disabled sticker to stare him in the face and remind him of his disability. More likely, if humanly possible, he will reject the easy option of parking right outside the store and strive

**THE BOTTOM LINE**

Some factors are beyond your control,
but **you** are the deciding factor.

instead to walk those extra few yards, stretching himself and facilitating the means of yet further advances in recovery. Remember, the muscles themselves are not damaged by stroke.

Three adverse factors occurring in the first few days of stroke are unconsciousness, urinary incontinence and deviation of the eyes to one side. The more catastrophic the stroke, the harder it is to recover – but even this is variable! There are numerous examples of stroke patients regaining consciousness and going on to make a sterling improvement in the months and years ahead.

The first 10 days, despite being volatile and difficult, often show the most rapid degree of healing. Brain cells which have died no longer have the capacity to recover, but others, just outside the area of primary damage, may only be temporarily malfunctioning due to leakage and swelling. In the aftermath of stroke, as these problems fade away and clear, surrounding and adjacent brain cells revert to normal functioning and the patient makes spontaneous improvement.

The next few weeks can also show spectacular gains as other undamaged brain cells in the vicinity of the stricken cells learn to mimic the actions of their predecessors. After that, although improvements can and will continue for up to three years, realistically, the rate of recovery begins to slow down.

The will to recover, as with the refusal to worry, is of supreme importance to all seriously ill patients. Some individuals simply give up and wait to die, or sentence themselves (and perhaps others) to a life of misery, when they might have had the capacity to do better.

Stroke is bound to put tremendous pressure on the relationship between patient and carer. A sense of humour is invaluable. If you can both see the funny side of efforts that misfire, this can ease the tension, speed recovery and bring you closer together.

# 5: Factors affecting the degree of recovery

> *It is a mistake to look too far ahead. Only one link of the chain of destiny can be handled at a time.*
>
> Winston Churchill 1874–1965

It is possible to recover all the physical damage due to stroke even if it was at first very severe. Hundreds of thousands of people have already done so, including myself. The widespread misconception that 'nothing can be done about stroke' is at last being swept aside as advances are made in prevention, acute treatment and rehabilitation.

Don't worry if you appear not to be the ideal stroke patient under the best of circumstances. There are pros and cons for us all. If you have a stroke when you are young, youth is on your side and you have a splendid chance of ultimately making a complete recovery. It can take longer to recover in old age but advancing years are accompanied by wisdom. Those patients who are neither young nor old have the best of both worlds. They retain the gift of comparative youth to fuel their recovery and a measure of maturity with which to mastermind their comeback.

I could scarcely comprehend the written word in the months directly following my second stroke. Now I can put together a book offering you guidance for your recovery. Amazing things can happen when you look for the positive in a bad situation.

## THE BOTTOM LINE

## Take one day at a time.

## What affects the degree of recovery?

- The amount of damage inflicted on the brain by stroke
- The area of the brain affected
- The age of the patient
- Early treatment in the specialized stroke unit of a hospital
- Guidance in practical stroke management and recovery of the type found in this book
- The patient's ability to relax, keep calm and not worry in the early days after stroke
- The availability of an experienced chartered physiotherapist
- The will to get well, as the greatest scope for recovery occurs soon after stroke
- A sense of humour
- The expectation of recovery as expressed to the patient by the consultant or doctor
- The support of family or friends or *someone who cares*
- A meaningful (perhaps new) purpose in life, no matter how modest
- The ability of both patient and carer to adapt to changing fortunes and difficult emotions
- The willingness of the patient to struggle and persevere for up to three years if necessary

# 6: Relaxation. Calm

> *… Like a ship that's rounded*
> *the cape, you will find yourself*
> *in calm water, the raging sea*
> *subsided, floating on gentle*
> *waves.*

Marcus Aurelius AD 121–180

In order to cope with stroke and recover, or to care for somebody who is in the throes of living that nightmare, the art of relaxation, remaining calm in a crisis, is beneficial to both parties. Prepare yourself for a relaxed and calming experience in a few moments from now. There follow some basic relaxation techniques that really work. They will bring you instant calm and you will be able to use them time and time again in the weeks and months to come. Every time you employ one of these simple remedies for the anxieties of life, you will find your state of mind eases more and more and that you are better able to cope, no matter what is happening in your life at the moment.

Those readers who have flown overnight with an oriental airline will remember the blissfully calming and relaxing touch of a moist hot towel pampering their face. You don't have to be 39,000 feet above to savour the ecstasy. Treat yourself now, before you read on. If you cannot, perhaps because you are confined to bed, promise yourself you will indulge at the earliest opportunity. After all, you are the most important person in your world. Don't you deserve a little luxury in your life? If you have just answered 'No', regard my suggestion as medicine and do it anyway!

Taking time to enjoy life's simple pleasures does not only improve our frame of mind, it can also help to encourage our bodies to the peak of health.

**THE BOTTOM LINE**

Every moment of calm is a step towards recovery.

The smell of roses can measurably boost the immune system and the accompanying feel-good factor can last for hours, according to ARISE, a group of scientists and academics dedicated to researching the health benefits of happiness. Its founder, Professor David Warburton, Head of Psychopharmacology at Reading University, writes:

> One study showed that recalling happy thoughts in a writing exercise led to a marked improvement in mood and a clearly increased level of immune response.

With the professor's words in mind, there is a wonderful exercise you can do using a rose and a glass of water. With one beautiful rose to hand (or *imagine* a newly-bloomed red rose in the cup of your hand) take a long, slow breath as you savour the scent and recall happy memories from the past. Further relax yourself by sipping water.

*And now to Paradise beach…* This next exercise is one of my favourites. Over the years it has successfully relaxed and calmed hundreds of my clients and now it is going to work its *guided imagery* magic for you. Initially, you will need someone to read the text on page 33 to you while you relax in bed (or in a chair) and close your eyes. Don't be afraid to ask.

With practice, you will find it possible to relax deeply and rapidly and return to reality refreshed and ready to face the challenges ahead. In time you will find that you can make it alone to Paradise beach without the need for anyone to read you the words.

*THE MIND*
*is its own place,*
*and in itself can make a heaven*
*of hell,*
*a hell of heaven.*
Milton 1608–74

## Paradise beach

… Close your eyes and become aware of your breathing. Take a few moments to settle.

Keep your eyes closed but imagine what you could see if you were to open them. Fix your mind on just one object in the room with which you are familiar and explore its shape… its texture… its contours.

Imagine now that it is melting but without any warmth or danger. Imagine it dissolving into white sand, crumbling under its own weight and becoming an assemblage of sand. Be aware that everything around your object is also crumbling into sand until you are left lying or sitting on an expanse of shimmering white sand.

You are on Paradise beach… a beach of soft, white sand. Towering behind you are palm trees gently swaying in the breeze. In front of you is the crystal-clear sea. You can hear the water lapping the beach and feel the warmth of the sun on your skin. There is a slight breeze keeping you at a safe and comfortable temperature all the time.

Be aware of the sky above you with its fluffy, cotton wool clouds passing overhead and away to the horizon. Feel your muscles relax and become more flexible as you lie or sit on this beautiful island where you are alone and undisturbed. You are happy under the sun and enjoying the peace and quiet of solitude with only the birds and butterflies to keep you company. Above the

**THE BOTTOM LINE**

There is a place on Paradise beach for you.

sounds of the sea, listen to the far-off cries of seagulls and experience the bliss of freedom from all your cares and worries.

If you want to you can stretch out on the beach and feel the warm sun on your body. You can move into the water and feel the gentle waves pulsating against your ankles. Feel the sun penetrate your body, reaching deep into your bones, loosening all your ligaments and tendons, filling you with a warm sensation, calming and relaxing you.

Now prepare yourself to leave this place and come back to reality. Keep your eyes closed. Take a last look around you, firmly establishing whatever you see on your consciousness, so that you can easily return here whenever you wish.

Slowly become aware of the sand around you reverting back into the shape of the object you originally fixed your mind upon. Without opening your eyes, visualize the rest of the room in which you are lying or sitting. When you feel ready, gently stretch your body and open your eyes. You are calmer and more relaxed than you were before.

# 7: What can the doctor do now?

*The art of medicine consists of amusing the patient while nature cures the disease.*
Voltaire 1694–1778

First, your doctor will want to ensure that the diagnosis of stroke is correct. If he has been called out to a patient who has suffered a major stroke, the chances are he will call for an ambulance at once. In my case, I was alone at home in my

## THE BOTTOM LINE

Medication may be necessary but time is the answer.

study and thoroughly exhausted and disoriented by the debilitating impact of stroke. Fortunately, my doctor's emergency number was logged into the top left-hand button of my autodialer. The telephone was on the desk directly in front of me. It took a great deal of effort and co-ordination to press that button and babble into the speaker, but I was rewarded with a doctor within minutes and an ambulance soon afterwards.

The prevention of complications is of particular concern to your doctor and these will be anticipated, diagnosed and treated. Complications are medical problems that are *not* recognized as an inevitable part of stroke illness itself. For example, paralysis is an integral part of stroke, whereas bed sores are not. The five most common causes of potential complication that your doctor will be seeking to guard against are listed below.

## Swallowing-relating complications

- choking
- dehydration
- starvation

## Paralysis-related complications

- shoulder pains or swelling of the hand on the stroke side
- injury due to falling over
- accidents due to reduced awareness of the affected limbs
- deformity of the joints

## Lack of mobility-related complications

- pressure sores
- chest infections

- constipation
- blood clots in the veins of the legs

## Mood-related complications

- depression

## Brain damage-related complications

- epilepsy
- burning pains in the affected limbs (rare)

---

### Medication

Your doctor will also monitor your blood pressure and possibly your cholesterol level. In cases of high blood pressure and hypertension – common causes of stroke – he will prescribe medication. Make sure you continue to take all medications prescribed until otherwise instructed. It could mean the difference between life and death. Aspirin is known to be effective in thinning the blood so that it passes through narrowed arteries more easily. You may be advised to take one or two low dosage (75 mg) tablets of soluble aspirin daily.

# 8: What can I do to help myself?

*Do what you can, with what
you have, with where you are
now.*

Theodore Roosevelt 1858–1919

The first task is to define exactly what can be done to stimulate recovery, then determine the priorities, breaking each one down into small, accomplishable steps. The most potent course of action is to follow the doctor's advice to the letter.

Patients who are fortunate enough to be granted access to therapists from one or more disciplines should attend at every opportunity to participate, pushing themselves as hard as they reasonably can.

In the days immediately following stroke, the majority of patients will be too dazed to think and plan with precision. They will need help and support from their carer in breaking down priorities into simple, manageable tasks. It is not by accident that the *bottom line* of text in this book is deemed to be comprehensible to almost all stroke patients, whereas the run of page text is more suited to carers and patients who are clearly on the road to recovery.

Time spent with patients within days of the occurrence of stroke, demonstrating how best they can help themselves, will reap dividends in the months and years ahead. Although patients can reasonably expect to go on getting better for up to three years, the greatest scope for recovery occurs soon after stroke.

At the earliest opportunity, encourage your patient to read *the bottom line* and comprehend it. The essence of each section is encompassed within those few words.

**THE BOTTOM LINE**

## Do your best. Summon the will to recover.

Without doubt, the single most effective thing that any stroke patient with the capacity to recover can do is to summon the will to recover. That one act, providing it is sustained, deeply-rooted and coupled with a willingness to struggle when the going gets tough, will hasten recovery in most cases of stroke. Without it, an army of doctors and a detachment of highly-trained therapists would labour in vain.

---

**Some patients condemn themselves to death**

Stroke illness, in many respects, is a most peculiar illness. The healing starts in earnest only when the patient will allow it to begin. Those with the capacity to recover who simply lie back and wait, without lifting a finger to help themselves, may ultimately condemn themselves to death or to life in a wheelchair. They will not recover as well as patients with similar deficits who make an effort to do whatever they can to help themselves.

---

# 9: Commitment and the will to get well

*Willpower can and should be considered a greater subject of pride than talent.*

Honoré de Balzac 1799–1850

OK, so you're in a bad way. Fortune has not been kind to you and, understandably, you take a dim view of being singled out for stroke when you would be much happier being fit and well. Furthermore, you've heard some horror

**THE BOTTOM LINE**

Start with a spark of commitment. Burning commitment and the will to get well will follow.

stories about stroke victims being disabled for life (only a minority of which are true) and others about patients dying in their hospital beds (only a minority of which are true). You're not at all sure that you have the will to get well and you have no idea where to find it. To crown it all, your doctor seems strangely reluctant to give you an absolute assurance that you will indeed get better.

When treating a complex illness like stroke, doctors are bound to be cautious in all matters of forecasting the likelihood of recovery. Doctors are medical people. They have no psychic powers and generally they are not in a position to judge the all-important will to get well of the patient.

You may remember the case of Christopher Reeve, star of the *Superman* films. He was thrown from his horse and paralysed from the neck down. What sort of response do you think he got from his doctors when he enquired if he would ever act again? He showed them!

## Commitment and the will to get well

Let's talk about two kinds of commitment: *intention-based* commitment and *burning* commitment. Intention-based commitment is something you manufacture in your mind. For example, *deciding to do more for yourself.* You might promise yourself, or your carer or a nurse, perhaps, that you will do more. You want to, you intend to, but still you are plagued with self-doubt.

This intention-based kind of commitment doesn't bring all the forces of the universe with it. But it is a wonderful place to start! Once you really get started, and strive to do more and more, then at some point you will experience a dramatic inner shift. Burning commitment will take over. This brings with it the power to achieve the seemingly impossible. It carries with it an unstoppable momentum, an unshakeable determination to get well.

# denial

# 1: Who cares for the carer?

*Hast thou no care of me?*

*Antony and Cleopatra* (Act IV)

William Shakespeare 1564–1616

Who does care for the carer? In close families and some communities the answer might well be different, but in the tough world that most of us inhabit, the straightforward reply in two little words is – *the carer*! In the first shock wave of stroke, it is natural to feel a rush of compassion (or guilt?) which can make the role of carer seem natural, inevitable and sometimes even desirable. In essence, however, the only reason for the unpaid carer to care that is sustainable in the long term is love. If your motive is genuine, your duty of care, however difficult, will seldom seem like penance, more a welcome opportunity to repay the patient for past kindnesses. Sadly, many unhappy carers care for all the wrong reasons, and in amongst their mountain of misery, patients can sense and resent it.

Becoming a carer means being there for the patient when it matters, arming yourself with relevant information (you are doing that right now) and being prepared to ask for and get the help and assistance both you and your patient will be needing in the very near future. Most important of all is the task of motivating the patient.

Many carers succumb to their natural disinclination to put any strain on the patient. This can have a disastrous impact on the chances of recovery. Stroke patients must be encouraged to exert themselves. Be subtle, if it's in your nature to be that way. Be patient and supportive while giving your patient enlivening tasks to accomplish and master. But if all else fails, when it is known that your patient has the capacity to do better, be absolutely resolute and make

**THE BOTTOM LINE**

*Use* the resource section at the back of the book.

it clear to your loved one that you expect co-operation. You don't want a help-less hulk on your hands forever; you want the patient to get better. Not least because your role as carer will come to a successful conclusion, and that's by far the best way to care for the carer.

# 2: Family

> *Even a happy life cannot be*
> *without a measure of darkness*
> *and the word 'happiness'*
> *would lose its meaning if it*
> *were not balanced by sadness.*
> Carl Gustav Jung 1875–1961

Older family members may well have been touched by tragedy before but younger ones are sometimes at a loss to know how to respond to a loved one with stroke illness. The advice that follows should help.

## What you can do for the patient hospitalized by stroke

- Just being there means so much to the patient. You don't have to talk all the time.
- Use touch and reassuring nods with a patient who has extreme difficulty in communicating.
- Sit on the stroke-affected side of the patient if possible.
- Talk to the patient, even if they are unconscious or asleep. This can be therapeutic for both of you and the patient may be able to hear and under-stand you.

- If you cannot visit, do write or telephone. When phoning, initiate most of the talking yourself and don't be put off if all you get for your troubles is the occasional grunt or groan. The patient would like to talk but may not be able to string words together or pronounce them properly. Things will get better in time, particularly with encouragement.
- Tell the nursing staff about any other medical conditions that you are aware of.
- Does the patient normally use reading glasses, dentures, hearing aids, etc.? Are they available? If not, can you help?

## How you can help care for the patient in hospital

- Watch what the nursing staff do and don't be afraid to ask 'Why?' *You need to know.*
- Once you have observed how a task is accomplished, ask the nurse if you can help.
- Take an interest in any medication prescribed for the patient. Be aware of what it is for, the instructions for taking it and any undesirable side-effects to watch out for.

## How best to cope with your own feelings of distress

- Talk things over with family and friends.
- When you come away from the patient, let your feelings out. Don't let pain and sadness well up inside you. Cry if you want to.
- If, after visiting the patient, you feel melancholy and drained, do something uplifting to raise your spirits. *Treat yourself*! You have just done something good and beneficial for someone else. Now do something enjoyable for yourself.
- We are all human. If, prior to the tragedy of stroke, you were unkind to the

**THE BOTTOM LINE**

Now is the time to forget past differences.

patient or simply neglectful and now regret your actions but you don't know how to put things right, ask by phone or letter for permission to visit the patient. Even if you are refused, as you may well be, the patient will probably be touched that you cared after all.

# 3: Friends

*A faithful friend is the*
*medicine of life.*
Ecclesiasticus 6:16

If you are a patient who has suffered a major stroke, you will soon find out for certain who your *real* friends are. You are in for a few surprises. Some delightful, some not.

Being a realist, I had expected to lose my fair-weather friends when the going got tough, and in that respect they did not disappoint me. What was surprising and tremendously sustaining through the difficult times ahead were the ones who were genuinely concerned about my change of fortune, all but three of whom I had previously regarded more as business acquaintances than confidants. They soon showed themselves to be loyal and unwavering friends. Hopefully, before long, if they haven't done so already, your true friends will make themselves known to you.

A word of warning, however. Whoever your carer is – spouse, partner, friend, relative or volunteer – do not let them do too much for you. 'Why not?' they may well ask. Your carer's willingness to help may actually undermine your recovery. Restoration of muscle control depends on stretch and strain. If the incentive to *move* those muscles is taken away (because your loved one or friend is doing everything for you) recovery is less likely.

**THE BOTTOM LINE**
## Someone to care can make a difference.

Help yourself to get well. Be grateful for the offers of help from your friends, but try to do as much for yourself as you possibly can. Accept assistance only for those tasks that you genuinely cannot manage for the time being. That way you will be placing yourself in the express lane of recovery and it won't be long before you are delighting everyone with a noticeable improvement in your condition.

And what happened to the rest of your lifelong circle of friends? You might wonder. Some of them genuinely can't cope with the enormity of your tragedy and wouldn't know what to say to you if they did visit. Others assume that you will have lots of well-wishers at your bedside and don't wish to burden you, and the rest either don't know that you are ill or don't care.

If you have no family or friends living nearby, ask the nurse to tell the local support groups that you would appreciate a visit from a volunteer visitor. Some people are born to be carers and would welcome the opportunity to pop in and see you.

# 4: All alone?

*On stage I make love to 25,000 people; then I go home alone.*

Janis Joplin 1943–1970

Patients who are alone in the world can hardly be expected to have a rosy view of potential relationships and how they might develop. Concentrate on getting well for now and consider yourself fortunate that you have nobody else to worry about. We will talk some more about the good things in life and how to get hold of them later in the book. Make no mistake, life after stroke can be exciting! But sometimes we have lessons to learn about ourselves first…

**THE BOTTOM LINE**

Reach out to your new life. *It may be better*!

Many years ago, when I was in my 30s, I was a partner in a magazine publishing house with offices in London and Spain. My secretary for five years at the London office was a most valuable member of my team. Whenever I walked into the office, she would immediately decipher my mood and determine, as she smiled and said, 'Good morning', whether or not that moment was the right one to present me with any bad news or tricky assignments. I always held her in high esteem (as indeed I still do), and several years after selling my interest in the business, I stepped out of a cab and there she was…

It was lunchtime, so naturally we headed straight for the nearest pub and got ourselves up-to-date with all the latest news and gossip. Just as we were about to leave, I couldn't resist the urge to ask her what she thought of me as a boss! At first she tried a touch of subtle diplomacy to side-step the question. I persisted, confident in my mind that working for me had been the happiest five years of her working life. Being me, I just had to hear it from her lips!

She sat upright and looked me directly in the face. 'Are you quite sure you want to hear this, David?' she said, sipping the last of her wine. Obviously, she wanted to tease me with some minor indiscretion, I thought.

'You are the most inconsiderate person I have ever worked for. If I hadn't been dating your partner in Spain, I would never have worked for you in the first place. Do you remember that day when I almost crawled into the office on my knees?' I remembered it well. 'I had a slipped disc and you gave me hell for being late. Do you want me to go on?'

This was not what I wanted to hear and it prompted me to reflect that maybe I had some work to do on myself. I never got around to it, of course, not until stroke time. That was the time when I got shaken apart and found myself with the need (forced opportunity?) to put myself back together again. Strangely enough, my relationships, business and personal, seem to function more smoothly these days. You, too, will have your own opportunities to develop your new life and relationships. Who knows what satisfaction you will attain?

# 5: Loss of faith

> *The most wonderful thing about saints is that they were human. They lost their tempers, got angry, scolded God... made mistakes and regretted them. Still they went on doggedly blundering toward heaven.*
>
> Phyllis McGinley 1905–78

Sometimes, when devoutly religious people meet unexpectedly with the tragedy of stroke, they cannot believe that their God would allow this to happen to them. At a time when they need their faith more than ever before, they lose it, becoming bitter and resentful, further compounding their feelings of loss and betrayal. Being undecided on all matters of religion, I concede that I am not the obvious choice of author to restore their faith. Nonetheless, I welcome the opportunity to try.

The mental response to suffering a stroke is fundamentally a grief reaction. The patient is mourning the loss of faculties, lifestyle and status. Grief, a natural human reaction to loss, is a process of adaptation and passes through a number of recognizable stages regardless of whether the loss is a loved one, amputation or paralysis. These stages include *alarm, shock, denial, anger, guilt, acceptance* and *adjustment*. Fifty per cent of patients who experience a major stroke (compared to one in five of the general population) also go through a period of *depression*. This is the time when faith can be severely tested, directly prior to the final stage of *wellbeing*, when all those years of belief prove to have real meaning for many.

## THE BOTTOM LINE

Could this setback be a test of faith?

Everyone – believers, non-believers and the uncommitted – has to find their own special way of coming to terms with stroke. For me, as I lay dazed and partly-paralysed in my hospital bed, I needed a reason for this improbability from hell. I stared up at the ceiling and imagined, without difficulty, one or two of my former business associates and my recent ex-wife smiling at my misfortune. I could almost hear the words, 'Good, he had it coming!'

From those early feelings of outrage was born **my will to get well.** Being bloody-minded and demanding, I vowed that recovery just wasn't enough. By the turn of the millennium (then, over four years hence) I had to be back on track and going somewhere.

I handled the injustice of stroke by convincing myself that it was fair retribution for my assorted sins of the past and drew comfort from the belief that 'I was getting mine now'.

This theory was severely tested the next morning when I had another stroke, this one worse and more disabling than the first. Angry, bitter, and confused, I reflected that maybe I had previously underestimated my little transgressions from the past.

I dealt with the 'smiling enemy bit' by thinking, **'I'll show 'em!'**

---

### A sense of purpose

The core texts of the world's principal religions recognize that the quest for happiness is not without its challenges and obstacles. The experience of fulfilment would seem to involve some kind of spiritual journey through life which at times appears almost to go beyond the limits of human emotion and understanding. Stroke is a tragedy by any standards, but much good can come out of it if we are persuaded towards a healthier way of life. Some people may see it as a signpost, a forced opportunity to do something else with their lives.

# 6: Sex

*The pleasure is momentary,*
*the position ridiculous, and the*
*expense damnable.*
Lord Chesterfield 1694–1773

Sex is probably the last thing on your mind in the immediate aftermath of stroke. But as things improve, when you begin to feel better... what then? There is no clinical reason for restricting or changing sexual activities following stroke. Many people believe that sex may precipitate another stroke but there is no evidence to support this. If you are worried, check with your doctor before resuming normal sexual activity.

Patients do change their pattern of sexual behaviour to some extent, possibly because they feel less desirable and less wanted. In some cases of stroke, damage may be sustained by those parts of the brain concerned with sexual responses, but it is important not to make rash assumptions about this. There are indeed many possible causes of loss of libido, some of which are remediable. Sensory nerve damage, following stroke, can also interfere with the sensation of sex, causing much of the physical satisfaction to be lost.

From a practical point of view, physical disability may make sexual intercourse more difficult than before. Increasing age also takes its toll on the physical ability to express sexuality. With or without stroke, older men worry about their potency and women about losing their attractiveness. But the notion that there is a corresponding decline in sexual interest is most certainly mistaken. The decline in sexual activity as we get older has perhaps more to do with loss of opportunity than lack of inclination.

A fairly common explanation for diminished interest in sex by stroke

**THE BOTTOM LINE**

## Proceed with pleasure.

patients is medication. Some types of drugs frequently prescribed to control high blood pressure will decrease the normal sex drive and interfere with sexual performance. Prozac, a highly-effective antidepressant, may also cause poor sexual performance. Sexual feelings do not disappear just because someone has suffered a stroke and may be disabled. The principal cause of difficulty with sex after stroke remains the psychological effect of the catastrophe on the patient. In the majority of cases, the remedy is, literally, in the hands of the partner.

Visual stimulation is extremely important to a patient's arousal. A depressed sex drive after stroke can be awakened by the sight of the partner removing their clothes – but you know all this! If it's the dance of the seven vests that turns you on, go for it!

After the trauma of stroke, nothing brings a man and woman closer than the act of making love. Caressing and foreplay are more important than ever. Naturally, care must be taken in positioning the side of the body affected by stroke. Later in the book *(see pages 100–117),* movement and positioning are addressed in both words and pictures.

# 7: Laughter

*Men will confess to treason,*
*murder, arson, false teeth, or a*
*wig. How many of them will*
*own up to a lack of humour?*
Frank Colby 1865–1925

Years ago, long before the first of my two strokes, I remember reading a quite remarkable book by the American journalist, Norman Cousins, titled *Anatomy*

**THE BOTTOM LINE**

## Comedy is medicine.

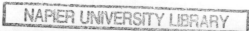

*of an Illness.* In it, he tells of his life-threatening and painful struggle with a spinal condition. He knew, from personal experience, just about everything there was to know about pain and he was aware that laughter had the power to release the body's natural painkillers, endorphins, into the bloodstream. One weekend, when the pain was monumental, he checked into a hotel, complete with a suitcase full of *Candid Camera* and *Marx Brothers* videos, and proceeded to test the therapeutic benefits of laughter. Cousins discovered that five minutes of spontaneous laughter (not polite, not restrained) gave him up to two hours of pain relief. And despite his chronic condition, he felt better about himself and life in general.

According to a Public Health study by Dr Lee Berk of California in 1996, laughter appears to boost the immune system. One hour of naturally-induced laughter significantly lowers levels of the stress hormones cortisol and epinephrine. It also stimulates and heightens the body's cells and antibodies. And who would deny that it can be instrumental in changing mood and banishing the blues?

Some people may regard laughter as inappropriate to stroke patients whose world has come crashing down on them. Nothing could be further from the truth. Laughter is essential in times of hardship. It helps us to survive the misery of incapacity by providing a distraction and the opportunity to let go. When we get better, laughter helps us to stay that way.

Stress management consultant, Robert Holden, who established the UK's first laughter clinic in 1992, believes that it is the emotional and social-bonding aspects of laughter which provide the real clue to its health-promoting qualities. He should know. In the first year of opening, 500 of the comically-challenged signed up for therapy!

I understand, from bitter experience stretching back to my teens, just how easy it is to become immersed in a downward spiral of depression in the aftermath of serious illness. When I was discharged from hospital after my second stroke, in a determined attempt to avoid the mistakes of the past, I asked to be taken home via a video store, where I stocked up on all my favourite comedies.

Every day, without exception, even when I felt miserable, I would force myself to watch at least two or three of them. Sometimes six! Sooner or later, despite my state, I invariably began to feel better. I rate laughter as one of the major contributing factors to my recovery. So, no matter how precarious your present circumstances, consider this page to be an open invitation to laugh whenever you want to. The people around you may think you're strange, but why should you care? **All you want to do is get better.**

# 8: Attitude

> *There is no cure for birth and death*
> *save to enjoy the interval.*
> George Santayana 1863–1952

Many patients make the worst of their stroke experience because they believe their affliction to be unjust. Serious illness, without exception, is always unfair. Life can seem like Russian roulette to the afflicted. Nonetheless, if you appreciate the force of George Santayana's words, doesn't it make sense to fight to overcome this injustice, rather than to be consumed by it? The difference is essentially a matter of attitude and your attitude right now and in the weeks and months to come will determine, to a large extent, whether or not you ride out this storm, your chances of recovery and your quality of life forever more.

There is no point in languishing in misery, because that type of negative emotion will sabotage your best chance of getting better. Our approach to recovery should be creative in finding new and different ways to combat paralysis and other deficits. At the same time we can rationally elect to adopt the

**THE BOTTOM LINE**

See if you can make someone smile today.

right frame of mind in which to benefit from the many treatments and therapies that will give our recovery a boost.

The major block to progress to most patients, given that stroke is a mean and disabling illness, is the trough of negativity that sometimes seems to be an integral part of the stroke package. How can patients isolate that part and divorce themselves from it? The solution comes in two easy and enjoyable parts. Try to master them both before you move on to the next chapter.

Admittedly, the joys associated with occupying a hospital bed or a period of rehabilitation are limited, but if you adopt the right attitude you will avoid digging yourself into an emotional trough. The best way to do this in your particular circumstances is to create, using your powers of imagination, an inner world in which fun and enjoyment are major elements. After all, your inner environment is the only one over which you exercise real control at the moment, and you alone possess the resource to rise above the negative situation in which you find yourself.

Building upon the previous chapter about the therapeutic effects of laughter, you may not be surprised to find that humour is the other part of the solution to breaking free of negative emotions. Like most things in life, it needs plenty of **practice**, but what a wonderful piece of homework you have before you, ladies and gentleman. A hundred lines with your stroke hand if you don't have lots of laughs in the coming weeks!

# 9: Treatment and care

*He that lives upon hope
will die fasting.*

Benjamin Franklin 1706–90

Whether you were admitted to hospital after your stroke or remained at home, there is likely to be a number of different professionals who may be involved in your care. Their individual roles in your recovery and rehabilitation are explained in greater detail elsewhere in the book. This section serves only as an introductory guide to the various professions that you may come into contact with. Bear in mind that there is still no specific medical treatment routinely available for many types of stroke. Once stroke has climaxed, the damage is done once and for all, and rehabilitation, not medical intervention in terms of an operation, is usually the way forward.

## General Practitioner

Your doctor will be responsible for your care if it was decided that you should remain at home. If you were admitted to hospital, your doctor will resume responsibility once you return home. Should you encounter difficulties in rehabilitation or have any worries about the effects of stroke, your doctor is the person to see. He or she can also refer you to other professionals.

## Consultant

In hospital you will be under the care of a consultant – a doctor specializing in one particular branch of medicine. He or she will decide whether or not you will benefit from an operation.

**THE BOTTOM LINE**

# Work **with** the professionals to **secure** your recovery.

## Surgeon

A minority of stroke patients undergo some form of surgery – usually involving the removal of a blood clot, the widening of a narrowed artery, or, in exceptional circumstances, the bypassing of a severely narrowed artery.

## Nurses

Hospital nurses play a major role in your assessment and rehabilitation. They are responsible for the day-to-day nursing and co-ordination of care. Tell the nurse if you have a problem. If you are unable to speak, don't worry, your nurse will know what to do. Community or district nurses work outside hospitals. They can visit you at home to assess your needs and they work closely with social workers, community nurses and care assistants to ensure your wellbeing.

## Physiotherapy

Most physiotherapists are located in hospitals or outpatient departments, although there are some who work in clinics, sports and health complexes and in private practice. Their role can be vital in getting stroke-damaged limbs moving again and they will advise and teach patients how to move correctly and exercise safely. Patients intent on optimum recovery would be well advised to put their heart and soul into every moment of physiotherapy treatment.

## Occupational therapy

Occupational therapists are your passport to freedom after stroke. They will help you regain as much independence as you can, motivating and assisting you to find new ways of coping with everyday activities such as getting washed and dressed and making yourself a cup of tea.

### THE BOTTOM LINE

Make everyone happy. Make every effort
to get better.

## *Speech and language therapy*

A speech and language therapist can help you overcome difficulties in communicating or swallowing. Their skills can seem almost miraculous to the patient struck dumb by stroke who, with time and effort, is gradually coaxed into communicating with the world once again.

## *Clinical psychology*

In addition to causing physical deficits, stroke can affect mental functions such as reasoning or memory. These malfunctions are usually only temporary and clear up in time of their own accord. In cases where difficulties persist, the clinical psychologist will assess these problems and, where practical, devise a strategy to help the patient overcome any outstanding difficulties.

# 10: Clinical assessment

*We should look long
and carefully...*
Molière 1622–73

Clinical assessment may involve one or more procedures to establish what medical treatment or rehabilitation strategy is most beneficial for you. The reasons for these investigations or tests are fourfold:

- To confirm that your symptoms were indeed caused by a stroke or mini-stroke.
- To establish what type of stroke you have suffered and why.
- To monitor your condition and decide how best to proceed.
- To determine the kind and degree of therapy or rehabilitation necessary in your case.

## Investigations your doctor may deem appropriate

1) BLOOD PRESSURE. It is likely that your blood pressure will be monitored regularly in the hours and days following your stroke.
2) BLOOD TESTING. There are a number of conditions that may have contributed to your stroke, including diabetes and blood cholesterol levels. Analysis of your blood can confirm or discount these.
3) ANGIOGRAM. This traditional method of obtaining an X-ray of the main arteries supplying the brain is called both angiography and arteriography. It involves the injection of a substance such as iodine (often wrongly referred to as dye) into the femoral artery in the groin, which

**THE BOTTOM LINE**

Clinical assessment can be your key
to rehabilitation.

shows up as opaque on an X-ray picture. This procedure, used to pinpoint a severe narrowing of an artery which may be suitable for surgery, is uncomfortable for the patient and, in itself, carries a very small risk of stroke.

4) CT (COMPUTERIZED TOMOGRAPHY) SCAN. This test is frequently conducted after stroke to provide detailed information on any structural changes which may have occurred within your brain. A machine takes X-ray 'slices' of the brain and can help to find out what type of stroke you may have experienced. Brain tumours (abnormal swelling) and haemorrhages (profuse bleeding from ruptured blood vessels) can also be identified from a CT scan.

5) CHEST X-RAY. This test investigates the underlying root causes of your stroke, such as a pre-existing heart or chest condition.

6) ELECTROCARDIOGRAM. This simple procedure measures the rhythm and activity of your heartbeat.

7) ECHOCARDIOGRAM. This cardiac ultrasound scanning device may be used to test for any underlying heart problems that might have contributed to your stroke.

8) ULTRASOUND. This Doppler (or Duplex) imaging technique is primarily used to detect arterial narrowing and is also ideally suited to patients who have suffered a warning *mini-stroke*.

9) MAGNETIC RESONANCE IMAGING (MRI). This highly sophisticated, state-of-the-art, brain scanning system gives a more detailed and accurate picture of the arteries than a CT scan.

# 11: Processes of recovery

*It is common sense to take a*
*method and try it. If it fails,*
*admit it frankly and try*
*another. ABOVE ALL,*
*TRY SOMETHING.*

Franklin D. Roosevelt 1882–1945

Some patients, including myself, recover almost completely from apparently devastating strokes, while others hardly manage to recover at all from comparatively minor ones. Why? It is true that age, the type and severity of stroke and even bad luck all have their part to play, but the most significant factor of all is the patient's will to get well.

## Processes of recovery

1) Natural recovery brought about by rest and the passage of time.
2) Reduction of swelling in the stroke-damaged area of the brain.
3) Learning alternative ways of coping.
4) Using other parts of the brain.
5) Limited growth of nerve axons in and around the brain-damaged area.
6) Increased sensitivity of existing neurons in the brain.
7) A surgical operation to implant live cells into the brain.

NATURAL RECOVERY is a partial process that occurs without any apparent intervention from either patient or doctor. The majority of stroke patients benefit from this phenomenon.

**THE BOTTOM LINE**

Keep on trying to reclaim your faculties until you do.

A REDUCTION OF SWELLING after 1–50 days allows the squashed brain to resume work.

USING OTHER PARTS OF THE BRAIN. All human brains, young and old, have spare capacity. Once an adult loses a brain cell it is gone forever, but during the regeneration process following stroke, undamaged neural circuits in the brain can be trained to take on new roles, for example, to control the muscle movements for walking.

LEARNING ALTERNATIVE WAYS OF COPING. Shaving or applying make-up with the good hand, instead of the stroke hand, is a typical example of rehabilitation.

LIMITED GROWTH OF NERVE AXONS can facilitate minor improvements to the brain's functioning by making contact with neighbouring cells.

INCREASED SENSITIVITY OF EXISTING NEURONS IN THE BRAIN is possible after stroke because the receiving part of a neuron can often compensate for reduced stimulation.

A SURGICAL OPERATION TO IMPLANT LIVE CELLS INTO THE BRAIN was first performed in the United States in 1999. The experimental operation was deemed by both patient and medical team to have been a complete success.

# 12: Surgery

*The world breaks everyone*
*and afterward many are*
*strong at the broken places.*

Ernest Hemingway 1898–1961

A minority of stroke patients may be suitable for some kind of surgery – usually involving either the removal of a blood clot within the brain, or the widening of an artery in the neck to improve blood flow. Four of the most frequently-performed operations to prevent the recurrence of stroke are briefly described below.

- Balloon angioplasty
- Carotid endarterectomy
- Clothes pegging
- Metal-coil treatment

## Balloon angioplasty

This operation, taking only an hour or two to complete, can be performed under a general anaesthetic and will, if successful, restore normal blood flow to a narrowed internal carotid artery. Balloon angioplasty is a preventive treatment – not a cure for a stroke that has already occurred. In this procedure a balloon on the tip of a catheter (a long and thin flexible tube) is inflated at the narrow section of the artery to widen it. Patients can expect to be sitting up in bed enjoying their breakfast the next morning and out of hospital in two or three days.

**THE BOTTOM LINE**

# Some stroke patients will benefit from an operation.

## Carotid endarterectomy

In cases where a critically narrow section of the internal carotid artery in the neck is detected in an angiogram prior to a large blood clot actually forming, carotid endarterectomy can significantly reduce the risk of stroke over the next two or three years. The artery is opened up with the patient under a general anaesthetic and the narrowed part is cleaned and cored before being closed. Again, the patient can expect to be out of hospital within a few days.

## Clothes pegging

Not a strictly medical term, but an accurate description of the way surgeons seek to prevent haemorrhagic strokes caused by rupturing bulges in a weakened section of an artery. Sometimes, as a result of prolonged high blood pressure, little balloon-like pouches can appear in the wall of an artery like the inner tube of a worn or damaged bicycle tyre. As the name implies, surgeons seek to close off the offending pouch with miniature 'clothes pegs' before it bursts. This procedure is performed under general anaesthetic.

## Metal-coil treatment

A less common procedure to the one described above is for surgeons to snake a catheter through the artery and place miniature metal coils into the bulge. This has the effect of preventing the bulge from rupturing or re-rupturing because blood clots round the coils to contain the bulge.

---

Do not feel disappointed if you are not offered an operation. The majority of stroke patients will not benefit from surgical intervention once their stroke has occurred.

# 13: Endurance and the willingness to persevere

*At 49 years of age, after my second stroke, I could no longer read or comprehend a news- paper. At 52, I wrote this book.*

David M. Hinds 1945–

My niece, Jane Fletcher, knows much about endurance and the willingness to persevere. While I lay ill in the John Radcliffe Hospital, Oxford, having been transferred from another hospital where I had suffered a second stroke within days of being admitted, Jane sprang into action. She decided to be the one to rescue her Uncle Dave.

At the time, she was a barmaid with three young children to feed and I had been the globetrotting chairman of a network of stress management consul- tancies. I was accustomed to life in the fast lane and my regular vacations in Rio; she was accustomed to making ends meet with difficulty. Although, prior to my subclavian bypass operation some months later to reduce the risk of yet another stroke, I was in no condition to help myself, the last thing I relished was early retirement in Jane's back bedroom.

She, on the other hand, was adamant that what I needed was a prolonged spell of life in the slow lane. She started a successful campaign to win approval from my family and friends and had me shipped to her home in Cornwall, knowing full well that I was likely to be the most unreasonable guest she had ever entertained.

**THE BOTTOM LINE**

# Nothing in the world can take the place of persistence.

We both laugh about my ill-humour now that I am better and living half-a-mile away. At the time it was no fun being unable to read or fully comprehend her little boy's *Thomas the Tank Engine* book. I remember the first time I was confronted with written words after my stroke. The word 'mother' was a mystery to me. Not only could I not pronounce it, I couldn't conjure up the significance of the word in my mind. I had to learn to read again.

I attempted every possible way of pronouncing each word until something in my damaged brain registered and I got a familiar image in my mind's eye. 'Mot-her' didn't ring any bells. Nor did 'm-other' but 'moth-er' – bingo! I had one of those. A nice one.

For the next few months, I spent an hour or two every morning trying to read children's books. I persisted, and in the end I made it to the very last page of *Thomas the Tank Engine*!

On the wall directly above my computer monitor is a priceless quotation by Calvin Coolidge. Whenever the words to write this book evade me I look up, read it and keep on searching.

---

### Nothing in the world can take the place of persistence

Talent will not; nothing is more common than unsuccessful men with talent. Genius will not; unrewarded genius is almost a proverb. Education will not; the world is full of educated derelicts. Persistence and determination alone are omnipotent.

PART FOUR

# anger

# 1: Stroke rage

*The greatest discovery of my
generation is that human
beings can alter their lives
by altering their attitudes
of mind.*

William James 1842–1910

How dare some phantom from hell, in the space of a few brutal but painless moments, penetrate my brain, paralysing my body on one side? What strange, sadistic force, I wonder, would rearrange my face so that one corner of my mouth was an inconvenient inch higher than the other, then transform me, an articulate person, into a babbling fool? Is this the devil's idea of Saturday night on the town?

Some patients, awakening from the nightmare of stroke to find that it has not ended, that it's taken them over, unleash their feelings of hopelessness and misery on those they know and love best. This nowadays can be called stroke rage and it must never be tolerated, not once. The energy from that outburst and any future eruptions must be redirected at the real enemy, stroke illness and the need to overcome its effects. Carers should try to arrest a display of stroke rage by diverting the patient's attention elsewhere. This works well providing the initiative is seized early and the patient taken by surprise.

Stroke rage is at the end of the anger spectrum. It is usually the result of mounting negative feelings caused by a succession of disappointments and setbacks and the realization that stroke will not simply fade away like flu. In much the same way as pressure building up within a pressure cooker, the moment comes when you have to let off steam. Unless the patient is actively committed

**THE BOTTOM LINE**

Go easy on yourself and your loved ones.

to a get well plan and believes that there is a genuine chance of recovery, stroke rage can take hold of the patient, momentarily blocking out all rational thought. This incites the patient to act solely on their emotions which, at that moment, are unpredictable. Fortunately, few stroke patients succumb to this level of emotional instability: it is a passing phase, disappearing completely within a month or two of onset.

It is often assumed by family and friends that hostile and sometimes petty behaviour is the direct result of brain damage. To a certain extent this may be true, but it should not be forgotten that stroke is a devastating calamity and much of the patient's puzzling behaviour is simply a natural reaction to what is a most distressing situation.

---

### Carer beware... seize the initiative!

- STROKE RAGE IS RARE BUT DON'T TOLERATE IT. MOVE THE PATIENT ON.
- Try to stop it by calmly directing the patient's attention elsewhere. This works well.
- It is more likely to manifest itself in patients who are not actively engaged in getting well or those who don't believe that they have a genuine chance of recovery.
- Be prepared! Have a surprise announcement up your sleeve at all times.

# 2: Bitter thoughts

*If we could read the secret
history of our enemies, we
should find in each man's life
sorrow and suffering enough
to disarm hostility.*

Henry Longfellow 1807–82

Stroke can strike anyone, even the young and healthy, at any time. Every year 15.3 million strokes occur worldwide and the number is steadily rising. The most frequent casualties are those at the height of their working careers and the retired. People, in the main, who have worked all their lives and had every right to look forward to a long and enjoyable retirement. If the person afflicted has a family, the loss of status as provider or contributor can be soul-destroying. No wonder then, when stroke knocks at the front door, bitterness creeps in round the back.

Men suffer strokes more than women. A difficult situation can be made worse by the patient's partner believing that they may have contributed to the onset of stroke by making excessive financial, social, or even sexual demands. Amid waves of guilt, partners recall troublesome times in the relationship when their own actions might have been unjustifiable and proceed to blame themselves for what has happened.

This is a frequent reaction among wives of hard-working, successful men who suffer strokes at the height of their career. Such a reaction is understandable but illogical. Who better to reassure readers on this important point than Dr R.M. Youngson, a Member of the British Medical Association and a Fellow of the Royal Society of Medicine. In his excellent book, *STROKE!*,

**THE BOTTOM LINE**

## Forgive and forget.

Dr. Youngson assures readers that strokes are not caused by hard work. Factors that can contribute to stroke are 'a lifetime of self-abuse, dietary over-indulgence, inadequate exercise, smoking and the inheritance of genes predisposing the recipient to cardiovascular disease. The tendency to build up stress by engaging in high-pressure work is not likely to be the result of a wife's urging, but will almost always be an inherent quality'.

Another area ripe for the fermentation of bitter thoughts is the thorny problem of legal responsibility. Stroke patients may well be people of wealth or influence, accustomed to exercising power but, if, through debilitating illness, they are unable to conduct their own affairs then clearly somebody else will need to do it for them. It is essential that whoever attends to the affairs should enjoy the complete confidence of the patient.

A word of warning. Just because the patient is unable to communicate easily or at all, it does not mean that there is nothing going on inside their head. It is perplexing to gauge the comprehension of an individual when the usual ways of communication are blocked, but be sure to give the patient the benefit of the doubt and seek their agreement in all matters concerning their future. Even when I was barely able to express myself or comprehend the written word, I knew what was going on.

# 3: Anger, hostility and tears

> *I was angry with my friend:*
> *I told my wrath, my wrath did end.*
> *I was angry with my foe:*
> *I told it not, my wrath did grow.*
>
> William Blake 1757–1827

We are all angry people – some of us just show it more than others. When we expect something and don't get it, when we are expecting nothing but get bad news, it disorientates us, making us feel irritated and distrustful. Without anger, happiness would lose all meaning. We need both light and shade to make our lives rich and colourful.

When stroke patients cannot manage the unfairnesses of life, they lash out and let everyone else feel a little of the rage that's going on inside them. There's nothing to be ashamed of in feeling angry at times, but when anger takes over and pervades every aspect of recovery, causing friction and hostility between patient and carer, you have to do something about it.

A major complication for carers when dealing with angry patients is that they cannot always be sure that the emotion displayed is the one being felt. The effects of stroke are so numerous and complex that sometimes it takes a skilled clinician to work out what the patient is really feeling. The patient may show all the signs of contentment while being miserable, or demonstrate furious anger while not actually being angry at all. Those of us who are not professionally qualified tend to take the signs of emotion at face value and it is difficult not to respond in the normal way. To someone trying only to help, an aggressive response from the patient is always hard to bear. I have been given strict instructions from my niece, who cared for me during much of my

**THE BOTTOM LINE**

Try not to bottle up your feelings.

convalescence, to 'put that in the book'!

It is in the nature of stroke illness for patients, no matter how out of character or unseemly it may be, to simply burst into tears. Crying is part of the recovery process and can be tremendously therapeutic. It demonstrates awareness and growing acceptance of the stroke phenomenon and is a healthy release of emotion. Very often, patients feel overcome by the need to cry their heart out and it can seem impossible to stop, no matter how hard they try, no matter how comforting and consoling their carer and friends may be. Although this phase in the recovery process is distressing for patient, carer and everyone concerned, it will eventually run its course. A major step forward is the likely result.

> No matter how you feel right now, *force yourself* to smile. If you can smile in the face of anger, you can summon the will to get well.

# 4: Using emotion to fuel recovery

> *Nothing contributes so much to tranquillise the mind as a steady purpose: a point on which the soul may fix its intellectual eye.*
>
> Mary Shelley 1797–1851

Anger is usually triggered by an event, a word, a person's behaviour, or our interpretation of any one of those things. It sets off our stress hormones, adrenaline, noradrenaline and cortisol, arousing tension in the body. Stroke patients, in addition to the run-of-the-mill provocations of daily life, often feel

**THE BOTTOM LINE**

When you're angry – try the mirror technique!

frustrated, misunderstood and restricted, even before someone comes along to upset them. They are angry with themselves for being unable to function as normal, furious at the outrageous misadventure that has caused them to be this way, less able to let off steam by traditional means, such as playing golf, walking or working in the garden.

Holding on to anger is dangerous to health. Suppressed or internalized anger can lead to high blood pressure, and that is not recommended for stroke patients who want to live. Accepting that it is essential to work off our anger, how do we do it when some of us are disabled, confined to our hospital beds, or otherwise indisposed?

The best way for stroke patients to deal with anger is to meet it head-on, in the mirror! Don't hesitate. The next time you are enraged, hold a mirror to your face with your good hand and confront your angry self. Don't look away from your image just because you are distressed or because half your face is paralysed, or both. Hold your nerve and continue to look. You will very quickly feel the urge to calm down if only because you (and everyone else) look ridiculous when fuming and angry. At this point in the exercise you may find tears welling up in your eyes. That's good. Already venom and anger are bailing out through the windows.

Don't stop yet, even though you are winning. Already you are learning to exercise control and damage-limitation over your anger. Now you must master the art of diverting that powerful emotion to a worthwhile cause: fuelling your recovery to health.

Position the mirror, or prop it up, so that your good hand is free. Now, using both hands if possible, or just your good hand if you prefer, gently try to manoeuvre your face into the pre-stroke position. Depending on the degree of paralysis, it might take much coercing and ingenuity to get what, at first, may be only a momentarily pleasing expression.

**Persevere, for you are setting in motion a chain of events which can eventually bring about a genuine improvement to your sense of well-being.**

# 5: Memory loss

*Forgetting is the great secret of
strong and creative lives.*
Honoré de Balzac 1799–1850

We all tend to forget things as we get older, but it's a fact of life that stroke patients are likely to experience more severe memory problems than others. Most patients gradually recover their memories in the weeks and months following stroke, and improvement has been known to continue for up to three years. The most effective way to combat memory loss and stimulate recovery is to get involved with an absorbing hobby or purpose. Memory is a complex process, but it has a knack of sorting itself out and functioning better when engaged in doing something enjoyable.

## Tips to encourage your memory

* Keep life after stroke simple for a while.
* Maintain a fixed routine for the basic chores of life, doing things at set times of day.
* Try to get into the habit of putting things away in the same place every time.
* If you have been prescribed a whole load of drugs and you have difficulty remembering when and what to take, ask your pharmacist to package them in 'blister packs' for you, which have the days of the week printed on them.
* Write your appointments and the day's *get well* exercises down in a large, page-a-day diary. If you cannot write, improvise with symbols or whatever you can manage.

**THE BOTTOM LINE**

# Many people recover their memories after stroke.

When something needs doing, try to do it immediately.

- If you have something important to remember, repeat it to yourself many times and then go over it in your mind at frequent intervals.

- Use simple prompts to jog your memory. For example, until my memory improved, I would leave letters to post in the hallway and documents for meetings in my briefcase. I would position the briefcase right up against the inside of the front door.

- Whenever you are introduced to someone new, repeat the name at natural points during the conversation and try to think of something familiar to associate with the name.

- Leave helpful little messages around the place. For example, if you have invited a friend round for dinner on Saturday, leave a note by the milk in the fridge saying something like 'TAKE CHICKEN OUT OF FREEZER ON FRIDAY'.

- Rediscover (or reinvent) your childhood. Play games! All sorts of games are good for recovery and some can sharpen the memory without any apparent effort. The game of Monopoly played an important part in my comeback.

# 6: Half-vision (hemianopia)

*Our life is what our thoughts
make of it.*

Marcus Aurelius AD 121–180

Vision is the primary sense that provides maximum information to the human brain. Approximately half of the nerves which carry messages to the brain about what is going on around us come from our eyes. Our brain interprets this information in a sophisticated and complex series of steps. Sometimes, when the brain is damaged by stroke, this complicated process can be interrupted, making the day-to-day living of patients afflicted by half-vision a real struggle.

The word hemianopia is Greek and it means 'without half vision'. Half-vision affects three out of ten stroke patients. Patients with this condition have effectively lost their sight from one side. A sufferer can have a meal put in front of them and can eat from only one half of the plate, being unaware that the other half exists.

It is a common misconception that you see things on your left side with your left eye and vice versa. In fact, what actually happens is that you see things on your left side with the right half of your left eye and the right half of your right eye. Correspondingly, you see things on your right side with the left half of both eyes.

Here is a test. Look at the page on your left. The one directly opposite this page with the number 76 printed at the top. If you cannot see it, you may have half-vision. If you are affected in this way, your carer should detach all of the pages from this book and place them, in numerical order, in front of you, slightly to the right of centre. That way, you will be able to derive full benefit from this book, not just half of it. Your carer should not feel guilty about

**THE BOTTOM LINE**

Improve awareness of the blind side by increasing eye movements towards that side.

splitting the book apart; a self-help book like this is to be devoured for its usefulness.

Although nearly half of all those affected do experience some spontaneous improvement in their field of vision, and a further nine per cent fully recover their vision, this remains a difficult problem to treat. The most promising attempts at treatment have involved training patients to improve their awareness of their blind side by enhancing their ability to make eye movements towards that side.

# 7: Visuo-spatial malfunctioning

*Never forget that the most powerful force on earth is LOVE.*

Nelson Rockefeller 1908–79

Certain types of brain damage can produce complicated disorders of spatial orientation. These can be difficult to understand, but are of enormous importance to those who are caring for stroke patients. Some patients neglect one side of their body (usually the left) and may even deny the existence of their own left arm. Occasionally, the patient's perception of their arm is so distorted that they believe it to be longer or shorter than normal, or covered in hair like a gorilla. In extreme cases, the patient will be absolutely convinced that the left arm belongs to someone else (a nurse standing nearby, perhaps), despite the indisputable evidence to the contrary.

The feeling that the left arm is indeed a foreign object may be so intense that the stroke patient actually attempts to throw away the offending arm,

**THE BOTTOM LINE**

You must try to adapt to unusual circumstances.

claiming that it is merely pinned to their body. Reactions like this appear to be completely irrational and may be mistaken by carers for psychiatric problems.

Patients with a severe disturbance of spatial function may be, for example, unable to draw symmetrical objects, such as a house or a clock-face, the left side of the object being usually less well drawn than the right. They are often unable to dress properly due to a difficulty in organizing their clothes. Some patients may attempt to put on a shirt or a blouse which is back-to-front and inside-out. Deficits of this nature are frequently referred to as perceptual problems or issues of neglect.

A problem which can be easily confused with visuo-spatial malfunctioning but is, in fact, a defect of motor programming, is known as apraxia. This is the loss of the ability to carry out familiar movements despite the absence of paralysis. For instance, a patient may genuinely be unable to stick out their tongue when requested to do so, but may have no difficulty with involuntarily licking their lips.

Apraxia is not the same as confusion. The vast majority of patients are confused and disoriented after stroke but this usually clears within a few weeks. Apraxia is a rare and more complex condition involving the inability to plan the necessary actions to transmit words. In severe cases both writing and speech can be affected and the patient with apraxia may not be able to speak intelligibly or at all. Progress is invariably slow. Advice and assessment from a fully-qualified speech therapist is essential. More specific information on a range of speech defects follow on pages 122–130.

# 8: Calming your emotions

*The important thing in acting
is to be able to laugh and cry. If
I have to cry, I think of my sex
life. If I have to laugh, I think
of my sex life…*

Glenda Jackson 1936–

'She felt her blood boil.' We all understand the cliché. What many of us don't realize is just how close to the truth sayings like this are. Our blood doesn't actually boil when we get mad, of course, but our blood pressure most certainly rises as we fume and seethe. Over time, with intermittent peaks of anger, like a boiler building up pressure, blood pressure keeps on edging up and staying up until stroke or some other health problem presents itself to those already at risk of arterial disease.

If we strip away all the niceties and do without the polite labels that doctors use, this is self-abuse. Let's find a better way to handle our emotions and redirect the rhythm and flow of our anger so that we no longer continue to damage ourselves and our loved ones. We can benefit from the wisdom and experience of others by putting into practice the two tried and tested techniques that follow, no matter how unlikely or preposterous they might seem.

## Old faithful

It is impossible to be both relaxed and angry at the same time. Give yourself a chance to respond imaginatively to situations that might otherwise make you lose your cool. Count to ten (silently, if you prefer) in a calm and measured

**THE BOTTOM LINE**

# Benefit from the wisdom and experience of others.

manner, taking slow, deep breaths all the way. Give yourself a helpful but challenging affirmation. For example, 'Right, now I'm under control, more or less'.

## *The stage prop*

For a nagging anger there is a method especially favoured by actors and actresses who have been driven almost to distraction by their directors. It is ideal for stroke patients who not only want to harmlessly work off their anger with someone who has enraged them, but who also wish to exercise their stroke hand. Take a nice fluffy bath towel between both hands and imagine you are using it to wring the blighter's neck. Go on, sink your fingers deep into the towel and twist! Think of the offender and extract your pound of flesh. You may find that your vengeance turns to tears. Don't be afraid; this means that your anger has been masking pain that is being squeezed out at last. This can be beneficial for you both, particularly if the subject of your emotions is a friend or a loved one. What's more, you've got a towel in your hands to wipe away the tears and embrace.

# 9: The inner strength to recover

*If a man lives without inner
struggle, if everything happens
in him without opposition...he
will remain such as he is.*

G. I. Gurdjieff 1877–1949

---

## COMMIT TO RECOVERY

HOT TIP... HOT TIP... Rather than tell yourself, 'I don't know if I can get better, so I can't commit myself to recovery', commit yourself anyway and then discover the therapeutic benefits to come. I assure you, during the course of my own recovery from stroke, I found the words of the following quotation by W.H. Murray to be truthful in every respect:

---

Until one is committed, there is hesitancy, the chance to draw back, always ineffectiveness. Concerning all acts of initiative, there is one elementary truth, the ignorance of which kills countless ideas and endless plans.

The moment one definitely commits, then Providence moves too. All sorts of things occur to help that would never otherwise have occurred. A whole stream of events issues from that decision, raising in one's favour all manner of unforeseen incidents and meetings and material assistance, which no man could have dreamed would have come his way.

**THE BOTTOM LINE**

## Until one is committed to recovery, there is hesitancy.

PART FIVE

# guilt

# 1: Guilt and resentment

*To be wronged is nothing
unless you continue to
remember it.*

Confucius 551–479 BC

Nice people, the caring, considerate type, suffer greater feelings of guilt than most, particularly the cold-hearted, selfish breed. Feelings of guilt have little connection with the actual degree of guilt, however judged. For instance, a serial rapist may feel no guilt whatever, whereas a patient incapacitated by stroke may feel guilty about the hardship and suffering caused to the family. Similarly, the spouse or partner may feel guilty over something said or done in the past, which has no actual connection with the patient's present condition. To make matters worse, guilt has a live-in partner, resentment.

'Look what a burden I have become!' bemoans the patient, already weighed down with fear. 'Just look at the worry, the expense, the embarrassment and all that unhappiness I am causing!'

At the same time, since guilt and resentment usually go hand in hand and most of us are less than perfect, the patient may well resent others of similar age and disposition who are enjoying the best of health.

The carer, despite all the love and care that is being given, may harbour feelings not unlike those of the patient.

'Did *I* cause the stroke by being too demanding?' (unearned guilt) or

'How can *I* have a life with all this unexpected responsibility to cope with?' (resentment).

Both patient and carer, who may genuinely love each other, are reacting to the same set of circumstances in similarly irrational terms from opposing perspectives.

**THE BOTTOM LINE**

## Let bygones be bygones.

Guilt and resentment are powerful emotions. They can be particularly difficult to wrestle with because they are, by their very nature, totally unreasonable emotions. They are partners in a dangerous mind game we play with ourselves. Their uncomfortable and energy-draining effects are the price we pay for not always taking a straightforward, realistic and balanced view of our own lives and the lives of those with whom we interact.

When you get right down to the very essence of guilt, it is anger directed inwards at ourselves. We are angry with ourselves for something we should have done or shouldn't have done. In any event, we are the ones that suffer most from our far from tender feelings because we are hell-bent on punishing ourselves – and we do.

Resentment is anger directed outwards at others but *we* are the ones that get hurt by our own negative, sometimes poisonous, thoughts and feelings.

In view of the fact that we shall be needing all of our emotional energy for worthy projects like getting well or motivating our partner to do just that, we are going to have to learn to let go of both guilt and resentment. They are luxuries you can no longer afford.

# 2: Self-doubt

*Every day, in every way, I'm getting better and better.*
Émile Coué 1857–1926

Visualize yourself almost completely restored to health. In your mind's eye, picture yourself without disability, enjoying life, living it to the full. You will recognize the familiar outer trappings of good health – the ability to walk to

**THE BOTTOM LINE**

Say it, write it, hum it, and try to **believe it!**

your local pub or club and enjoy drinks and a chat with old friends, the free-dom to travel as far as your finances will stretch, the joy and excitement of sex, the satisfaction of participating in your favourite sport or pastime and the sheer delight in spending time with loved ones.

The important thing is to imagine what it would be like to be well again. Do not think about it laboriously like mental arithmetic. Conceive it, look at it, touch it, smell it, listen to the sounds of laughter and happiness. Try to believe that you can be a part of it, now that you are connecting with your inner self.

I'm just guessing at your ideal lifestyle, of course, but the chances are you may have some way to go before finding it. Most of us are simply not there yet! Quite possibly, you still feel exhausted from the upheaval and trauma of stroke and you don't believe for one minute that you can get better. How can you be expected to believe in your own recovery when, understandably, you are so full of self-doubt you're not even sure if you'll be able to make it out of bed in the morning?

Given the capacity to recover, do those who have suffered a severe or dev-astating stroke have any realistic hope of getting better and regaining mobility? The answer, in the vast majority of cases, is a resounding YES. Take my own recovery as an example. I had to work at it for the best part of three years to get a satisfactory result (stepping on a few uncharted mines along the way) but there is tremendous satisfaction to be had in going after something we really want. Think back to your courting days! And three years is nothing: a brief jail sentence; the time it takes to complete a course of study. For the most glittering of all prizes, the chance to win back our health, are we not willing to serve a lit-tle time? No matter how undeserved.

Yes, you may say, but how do I get from where I am, this awful mess I'm in right now, to where you are, or somewhere equally pleasant? Just like you, I had my share of self-doubt, plus so many setbacks to my recovery that I was frequently disheartened. Between stroke and recovery lies a fair degree of hard work. If you are willing to put in the effort, the chances are you'll make it.

# 3: Personality change

*In times of great stress we are revealed in our true personalities.*

Shirley Jackson 1920–1969

'There's an ocean between us,' exclaimed one carer, a professional singer. 'It's as if he's a completely different person from the man I married! Will I ever get back that loveable rascal who used to drive me to distraction until that night when he was paralysed by stroke?'

Variations on this theme are all too frequent after loved ones have suffered a severe stroke, but in many cases the change in personality is not necessarily permanent and, following a transitional period, the change can ultimately be for the better. My closest friends say that I am more considerate and humane than I was before my strokes.

In certain cases of stroke, the physical damage, the psychological trauma, the stress of major upheaval and incapacity, or a combination of all three, can cause patients to be revealed in their true personalities, or with aspects of their personality altered. Sometimes, personality traits, over which patients exercised restraint prior to stroke, assume free rein. For example, a woman who had never suffered fools gladly who, in the past, had simply walked away from trouble, might become confrontational and abusive. A quiet, obliging sort of chap, who occasionally bit his nails, now becomes obsessed with them, to the disgust and annoyance of those around him.

Understandably, few adults, particularly those who have already suffered so much, appreciate having their lives directed for them and there can be a tendency in rehabilitation to become awkward and stubborn. This is demoralizing

**THE BOTTOM LINE**

# The change need not necessarily be for the worse.

for the carer, but it is self-defeating for the patient: the optimum chances of recovery are being thrown away.

By far the most productive times for getting back to normal are, in order of potency, the hours, the days, the weeks, the months, and then the first few years after stroke. Every effort the patient makes during these opportunities for convalescence will ultimately translate into how much, or how little, deficit remains for life.

The saddest thing about stroke is that your nearest and dearest can help but they can't enter into the struggle. No one but the patient can win. The most useful thing the carer can do beyond giving practical and emotional support is to get the patient genuinely interested and involved in their own future. That way the negative aspects of a change in personality can be minimized and, quite possibly, surmounted.

# 4: Stroke personality

*What a wonderful life I've had!*
*I only wish I'd realised it sooner.*
Colette 1873–1954

Medical research establishments around the world have carried out extensive studies to establish whether or not there really is such a thing as 'stroke personality': people, by nature of their personalities and behaviour patterns, who are more prone to stroke illness than others. Much of the research material available is interesting but inconclusive. However, I would suggest that we take note of research into stroke illness from countries as diverse as Sweden, South Korea and the USA on the topic of 'Type A' personality, that is the competitive, go-getter type of person.

THE BOTTOM LINE

# Do you have anything to learn from the research on the next page?

In the course of preparing for this chapter, I began to recognize myself (my pre-stroke self) from a pattern of behaviour that was described as dangerous to health and likely to lead to serious illness. After the trauma of two strokes, I found it relatively easy to make the necessary changes to avoid a third! Without drawing any conclusions, I would like you to see if there are any similarities between your own personality and the material that follows.

Personality can be reliably assessed by means of psychological tests, the most comprehensive of these being the 'Minnesota Multiphasic Personality Inventory–2' (MMPI–2). Developed by the University of Minnesota using a sample of 1,138 males and 1,462 females, this is a test in which participants are required to tick 'true' or 'false' to more than 500 statements. From an analysis of the responses, a remarkably accurate and detailed study of personality can be obtained.

Tests indicate that Type A people should look very closely at some aspects of their personality. For instance, those people with high hostility ratings are more likely to develop arterial diseases such as stroke or coronary thrombosis than those with low hostility ratings. Hostility is generally characterized by those who demonstrate their competitiveness and impatience with others by aggressive behaviour.

Studies at Duke University in Durham, North Carolina, suggest that Type A personalities who consistently bottle up their feelings of aggression are at even greater risk of arterial disease and stroke.

More recent investigations into Type A behaviour at Ulsan University, Seoul, South Korea, suggest that high and prolonged feelings of tension may be an independent risk factor for stroke.

Findings from a 1998 study of hypertensive men at high cardiovascular risk at University Hospital in Gothenburg, Sweden, concluded that patients with low self-esteem were more predisposed to future stroke than those with a higher sense of wellbeing.

Do you recognize yourself in any of this? If you do, perhaps a chat with your doctor or a stress counsellor is in order.

# 5: Tiredness and lack of energy

*Brain work is tiring; using
one's imagination is not.*
Enid Blyton 1897–1968

One of the maddening stings in the tail of stroke is how easily patients can become exhausted after comparatively little effort. Tiredness and lack of energy as a result of stroke is not necessarily a passing phase. Although I find I have far more energy now than in the first year of illness, even to this day I find it necessary to take a nap in the afternoon in order to make it through to the end of the day.

Almost everyone who has experienced stroke, however mild, suffers from tiredness and lack of energy to a degree. For many, the problem is confined to the initial period of recovery and begins to ease after a few months. For others, exhaustion can be a persistent problem affecting the patient's day-to-day life for years to come.

The only effective answer I have found is flexibility, to strive hard and resolutely in rehabilitation, then to rest straight afterwards, whatever the time of day.

Regardless of whether I have a speaking engagement in the evening, or I am simply meeting a friend for a chat, I always organize my affairs so that I get a siesta first. Otherwise, my voice begins to sound slurred as if I am drunk (when I'm not!) and my concentration goes out of the window. On the few occasions recently when I have been foolish enough to allow myself to get over-tired, I begin to feel the tell-tale sensations of nightmares past, the heaviness of hand and that prickly feeling on one side of my face, particularly around my mouth. No matter what I'm doing, I stop. So should you.

### THE BOTTOM LINE

# Push yourself hard, then have a siesta at any time.

It is not surprising that patients experience extreme tiredness in the weeks and months directly following stroke. After all, this is the time when your body is doing its best to heal and you are putting tremendous effort into master-minding the best possible recovery available to you. Some patients feel that physiotherapists and other therapists involved in their rehabilitation are work-ing them too hard, but they are invariably mistaken. The caring professions have only their patients' best interests at heart. They know exactly how hard to push in order to get results and when to stop.

---

**Tips for coping with exhaustion during rehabilitation**

- Rest before and after all rehabilitation sessions.
- Practise the new skills you have learned in therapy at times of the day when you feel most active. *Try to enjoy what you are doing!*
- Be patient and keep trying when it takes you a long time to relearn lost skills after stroke.
- If you should feel agitated or impatient with yourself during therapy, wind down and relax afterwards to your favourite piece of music.

# 6: The chances of survival

*Die, my dear doctor, that's*
*the last thing I shall do.*
Lord Palmerston 1784–1865

You will increase your chances of survival and ultimate recovery from stroke if you adopt the principles and recommendations for lifestyle changes described in this book. I say this with absolute conviction, the conviction of someone who has suffered like you are suffering, experienced what you are experiencing, encountered setbacks similar to yours and succeeded in regaining my health by these methods.

One question I am often asked is this: 'What is the secret of your recovery?' My reply never varies. 'Constancy to purpose.' Every part of my being was attuned to getting better.

Some stroke patients firmly believe they are doing all they can to regain their health. The test is *what are they doing to make that happen?* Are they actively involved in their own healing? If they were addicted to nicotine before their stroke, have they given up smoking completely, for example? The answers to these and other pertinent questions are not always as straightforward and encouraging as one might expect considering that survival from stroke is by no means automatic.

Survival and recovery are not, of course, entirely in the hands of the patient. But to a much greater extent than some stroke patients realize, their chances of a meaningful and active future are often up to them. We all, to some extent, have choices to make about our daily lives and the overall quality of them. Many patients choose by default – they choose by not choosing to change – and carry on with the bad habits of the past which may have

**THE BOTTOM LINE**

# The chances of survival from stroke are increased when the mind has a steady purpose.

contributed to stroke illness in the first place.

No matter what your ideological or religious beliefs, accept stroke (now that it is a part of you) as a test, an opportunity to rise above your shortcomings and reach for your finest hour. In my experience of putting myself back together again, I believe that once you are irreversibly committed to a worthwhile course of action, regardless of the difficulties ahead, all sorts of fortuitous happenings and opportunities come into play to help you along the way. The chances of survival are increased because there is no longer room in your mind for negativity and doubt to take root.

Before you turn the page, give some thought to your own purpose in life. Don't dwell on the lost opportunities of the past. Concentrate on what will give you satisfaction in the future. Fate has delivered you to a crossroads. You are there now. Bearing in mind that you are never too old to recover from stroke, will you take action to increase your chances of survival, or will you choose by default?

# 7: Goodbye to guilt and resentment

*Life teaches us to be less harsh
with ourselves and with others.*
Goethe 1749–1832

The mind is a marvellous filtering mechanism, and in this section we shall learn to use it to say 'GOODBYE' to the negative effects of guilt and resentment, thereby boosting our chances of recovery or excelling in our role of carer. There is a bonus for mastering the simple technique on the next page – the rest of your life, no matter what your circumstances are right now, can be more enjoyable and less painful than before.

## THE BOTTOM LINE

You are now free to enjoy the simple pleasures of life.

Our mind is constantly sheltering us from huge amounts of information. If it didn't, we would go mad because we can't possibly pay conscious attention to every single detail being collected by our five senses.

Without moving them, be aware of your lips. Were you aware of them a moment before? Probably not. The sensation was there, but your mind filtered out the information because you had no need for it. Had you been just about to kiss the person of your dreams, the sensation of your lips would have been foremost in mind and this book would be instantly forgotten.

What happens with guilt and resentment? Why do we become engulfed in waves of hatred for ourselves and others? How does that fearsome combination get a hold of us and then go on to penetrate and poison our innermost feelings? How does it all start?

With just one thought. Nothing more! Your mind had been successfully filtering out such negative emotions while you were actively engaged in doing something else, but once your attention had been grabbed by a pang of guilt or a perceived injustice, the demon and its spiteful playmate, resentment, went to work on your feelings, changing them and making you angry and bitter. You, in the meantime, not only rolled over and let them make you miserable, you entertained them as well: you gave them food for further thought!

Now that we know how not to do it, we can get it right for ever more. Don't dwell on those negative and self-destructive thoughts in future. When they come, as they will, simply say 'GOODBYE' and *think of something else.*

Refusing outright to dwell on feelings of guilt and resentment by switching your mind to something else, like just about everything else that is worth striving for in life, takes time, effort and constant practice before success can be achieved. Compared with the many trials and impediments to securing a measure of satisfaction and peace of mind in life, is not this one straightforward but repetitive technique worth adopting for your own personal benefit? Now and forever more.

# 8: Halfway house

*Perhaps the most valuable
result of all education is the
ability to make yourself do the
thing you have to do, when it
ought to be done, whether you
like it or not.*

Thomas Henry Huxley 1825–95

---

CONGRATULATIONS TO BOTH PATIENT AND CARER!

---

Despite tragedy, bad luck, and the many and varied setbacks and hardships of your misfortune, you have made it to the halfway point of this book. This, I know, from my own bitter experience of learning to read again after stroke, can be a major achievement.

Before moving onward to greater recovery and the remaining chapters, a **halfway house** celebration is in order. Relax and savour your achievement so far. Reach for a glass of champagne if that is possible. If you are in hospital, ask the nurse to pour you one (point to the word in bold type that follows if you cannot speak: **champagne**). Admittedly, you may not get it, but you surely will be rewarded with a warm smile and a cup of tea. You can still celebrate your achievement in your own private way. Never give up hope of achieving the best possible recovery available to you until you achieve just that.

**It is worth struggling for. You can be happy and contented after stroke.**

**THE BOTTOM LINE**

Well done! Already you are halfway through the book.

# PART SIX

# acceptance

# 1: Physiotherapy

*All our talents increase in the
using, and every faculty both
good and bad, strengthens
by exercise.*

Anne Brontë 1820–49

Expert advice and initial guidance from a physiotherapist is the key to maximum recovery of movement. A qualified physiotherapist has specialized knowledge about the body in motion and the stresses and strains upon it. Regaining the power of movement after stroke can only be achieved by pushing the body beyond its current limits. Understandably, many patients feel sorry for themselves and just want to be left alone in bed.

Lying in bed for long periods is dangerous to health. Although stroke patients do need plenty of rest, they should be encouraged to stretch themselves in the interest of regaining mobility. In the absence of a physiotherapist, a trained nurse will know how to get the patient moving safely. The essential thing to remember is that the patient *must* be placed in the correct position for movement. Learning to walk again is no easy business.

In an ideal world, a physiotherapist should be on hand soon after stroke. In reality, this is the exception, not the norm. Physiotherapists are very much in demand and patients may experience some delay, no matter how great the need. Don't give up! Keep on to your local health authority, hospital or community health centre.

Pages 100–118 contain step-by-step guidelines and illustrations for positioning seriously ill patients for movement after stroke. These will be of particular importance to you should that responsibility fall to yourself.

### THE BOTTOM LINE

# Be advised by a physiotherapist then **exert yourself.**

Aftercare for stroke patients is improving, and more physiotherapists are being recruited and trained. It can be helpful to show this edition of *After Stroke* to your physiotherapist and other health professionals. They will, in all probability, be conversant with the philosophy behind the book and the principles of maximum recovery that you are following. In view of their extensive training and experience, they may wish to recommend some additional or alternative strategies for you. Trust them, and put your personal effort and perspiration behind their expertise and judgement.

## *You need to know:*

*   Expert advice from a physiotherapist is the key to maximum recovery of movement.
*   Lying in bed for long periods after stroke is dangerous to health.
*   It is essential that the patient is placed in the correct positions for movement after stroke.
*   Checking posture in the mirror helps the patient to reinforce good symmetrical stance.

---

**Patient overweight?** *Carer beware*

*   An overweight stroke patient will often have a poor power-to-weight ratio i.e. much weight but little strength to move it.
*   Inactivity causes the muscles to waste away, reducing strength and impeding recovery. Although this applies to all patients, the implications are more serious for overweight patients who may never walk again after stroke unless they slim down.

---

# 2: Starting to move after stroke

*When she raises her eyelids it's
as if she were taking off all her
clothes.*
Colette 1873–1954

It is not always possible for the patient to move or stretch muscles and joints freely after stroke. This means that a limb may remain in one particular position all the time. As a result, the muscles and ligaments gradually adapt to maintain the limb in that position. If this is allowed to continue, the soft tissues become permanently shortened which then limits movement. This undesirable condition, known in medical terms as a 'contracture', can also be caused by muscle 'spasm' (also known as 'spasticity') which pull the limbs into a bent position.

---

**To avoid complications, carers should ensure that the patient:**

A) Changes position regularly.
B) Adopts resting positions which stretch the joints and muscles and support the weak side of the body.
C) Assumes the *correct* position for movement and relaxation as shown in the illustrations on the following pages.

---

Damage in stroke occurs only in the brain. Nothing at all has happened to the muscles themselves or to the nerves from the spinal cord. All these are intact and able to function. Even the connecting nerve bundles in the spinal cord are

**THE BOTTOM LINE**

# Beware spasm and abnormal positioning of deformity.

intact. The only thing wrong is that the nerve bundles passing down through the substance of the brain from the surface, whose job it is to tell the spinal nerves to stimulate the muscles into contraction, have been interfered with by stroke.

When the nerve impulses from the brain are absent, or abnormal, the lower nerves tend, after a time, to act on their own. Muscles affected are not only unable to perform voluntary actions at will, but can go into uncontrollable contraction on the slightest stimulus. To ensure that stroke patients are correctly positioned for movement so that spasm cannot be allowed to pull the body into an abnormal and fixed position of deformity, this section, and the following six sections on movement, are supplemented by illustrations provided by The Stroke Association in London.

If you have any worries, please consult your doctor or a chartered physiotherapist before embarking on any activity described in this book. The Stroke Association, myself and my publishers cannot be held in any way responsible for injuries or health problems caused by undertaking activities described in this book.

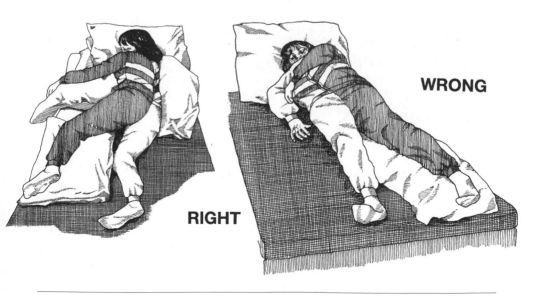

RIGHT

WRONG

FAMILY MEMBERS AND THOSE NEW TO THE ROLE OF CARER, MAY FIND IT HELPFUL TO BEAR THE FOLLOWING GENERAL POINTS IN MIND.

- Rather than attempt to lift someone or take the strain by yourself, try simply to assist the patient's movements.
- Before you begin, make sure that you both know what you are going to do and how you are going to do it. It can be helpful if you take the lead by giving the instructions during the movement. Agree in advance, with the person you are helping, that you will do this.
- Remove any obstacles before you start and get everything you need close to you.
- Wear flat shoes (e.g. trainers) and loose clothing which will not restrict your movement.
- Get as close as possible to the person you are helping.
- Always point your feet in the direction in which you want to move. Keep them about hip distance apart.
- If you should need to turn to complete a movement, take a step in that direction rather than twisting. It is essential that you do not twist. Twisting and bending at the same time puts a huge strain on your back.
- Use your legs as much as possible to avoid straining your back. Keep your back straight and bend at the hips and knees.

## Correct posture in bed

1) The best position for the patient to adopt is lying on the unaffected side because it keeps both shoulders and hips in the correct position and makes it easier to support and stretch the weak arm and leg. It is always beneficial to have pillows supporting the patient's head.
2) Correctly position the hips as on the left of the previous page. The hip on the weak side should be tilted forwards to prevent the patient from rolling

back, with the weak leg bent and supported by a pillow. The unaffected leg, which is underneath, should be almost straight.

3) By stretching the weak arm out in front and resting it on the pillow, the weak shoulder is being correctly supported. If the patient prefers, the elbow of the weak arm can be slightly bent. Rest the fingers of the weak hand so they are flat on the pillows.

4) Pillows behind the back should help the patient stay in a good resting position. The pillows will also help keep the weight of the body forward.

5) Check that the patient has not rolled and assumed the *wrong* position as illustrated on the right-hand side of page 101.

# 3: Changing position in bed

*U-turn if you want to.*
*The lady's not for turning.*
Margaret Thatcher 1925–

At the onset of stroke, muscles in the face, trunk, arm and leg on one side of the body are weak and lax. The affected side can be either the left or the right. In most cases power gradually returns, first to the leg and then to the arm. However, unless the limbs are placed in the correct position and are frequently put through a range of movements, there is a danger that they may stiffen and become unusable. This is why it is essential to maintain the limbs in the correct position, thus allowing recovery to take place over time.

The simple rule is to let the leg bend but to keep the affected arm straight. It is also vital to treat the body as a whole, not just the paralysed limbs in isolation. The position of the patient's head is of paramount importance. It has a

**THE BOTTOM LINE**

# Maintain paralysed limbs in the correct position.

great influence on the severity of spasm, should one occur. For instance, if the head is turned towards the weak side, the amount of spasm will be less. If turned away from the paralysed side, spasm will increase. Many stroke patients have a tendency to shy away from the affected side of their bodies and this tendency should be gently corrected whenever possible by the carer.

## Back pain

Weakness of the back muscles, as a result of stroke, can sometimes cause the recurrence of back problems such as arthritis or a slipped disc. Pain can also occur following muscle spasm, or because the weakened muscles no longer support the back properly.

---

**Ways to reduce back pain**

- Gentle heat can help to ease muscular pain. A hot water bottle (wrapped in a towel) can be effective but it must be used with care, particularly if the weak side is numb.
- Manipulative physiotherapy, acupuncture or osteopathy can be helpful for some patients.

---

## Shoulder pain

Shoulder pain is fairly common. Muscle weakness after stroke means that the shoulder joint on the weak side is no longer sufficiently supported. There is a risk that the soft tissue around the joint can become 'nipped' between the bones, causing inflammation, pain and damage. Take note: if a particular activity or movement causes pain, then stop immediately.

Lying on the back, except for short periods to relieve discomfort, should be discouraged because it can lead to poor positioning of the shoulder and hip on the weak side. Getting sufficient rest, however, is also important for the well-being of the patient, thus the illustration, at the top of the next page, shows the correct position for lying on the back, should that position become unavoidable.

---

**Ways to prevent shoulder pain**

- The stroke patient's arm should never be lifted by the hand.
- Avoid pulling on the weak arm at all times.
- Take great care to ensure the weak arm is always well supported.
- Never hold a stroke patient under the armpit when assisting them to get up from a chair.

---

Lying on the weak side in bed can be uncomfortable. If the weak shoulder is painful, it is better to avoid this position. If, however, this is the only position your patient finds acceptable, observe the correct position illustrated at the centre of the next page.

**Avoid the potentially harmful position shown at the bottom of the next page.**

## Lying on the weak side in bed

- Make sure that your patient has not rolled over onto their back. Pillows tucked behind the back should help maintain a good resting position.
- The weak arm and shoulder should be eased forward to ensure the arm is not trapped under the body. The weak arm should be turned upwards.
- The weak hip should be straight, so that the thigh follows a line straight down from the body. However, the lower part of the leg needs to be pulled back a little so that the knee is slightly bent.

• Finally, the unaffected leg should be pulled forward, with the hip and knee bent and in front of the weak leg, and supported on a pillow.

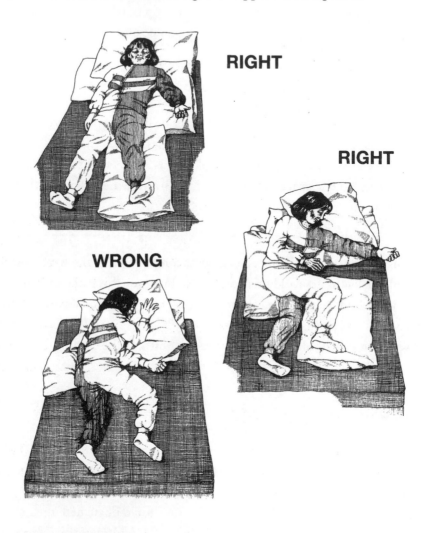

**RIGHT**

**RIGHT**

**WRONG**

# 4: Sitting up in bed

*Whatever you can do, or*
*dream you can, begin it.*
*Boldness has genius, power*
*and magic in it.*
Goethe 1749–1832

The first step towards getting out of bed is sitting up, but it is not a good position to adopt for long because there is a tendency to slump sideways. This may be uncomfortable and can make breathing more difficult. Sense of balance is often impaired after stroke and it is imperative that the patient should not be left alone in a new position until it can be safely maintained for a reasonable length of time.

It is usually easier to carry out activities such as eating, reading or watching television while sitting in a chair where a good resting position is easier to achieve. Should it be necessary to use a bedside table, be sure to position it on the patient's weak side, *not the unaffected side.* Although the spine must not be allowed to take on a permanent twist, it is nevertheless important that active voluntary movement towards the weak side should be encouraged. This discourages and minimizes spasm, advocates recognition of the weak side of the body and greatly assists the process of rehabilitation.

The correct way to sit your patient up in bed is illustrated on the next page, marked 'RIGHT'. (The wrong way is also shown, marked 'WRONG'.)

1) Sit up straight, with the buttocks as far back as possible.
2) Use pillows to support the back to avoid a half-lying, slouched position.
3) Weight should be evenly spread over both buttocks to prevent leaning to one side.

**THE BOTTOM LINE**

# Lying in bed for long periods is dangerous to health.

4) The body, *not* the head, should be turned if reaching towards a bedside table.

5) Support the weak arm on pillows, beside and slightly in front of the body, with the hand pointing forwards and fingers in a straight position.

6) Support the weak leg with a pillow under the thigh, or against the outside of the thigh, to help prevent the weak leg from turning out.

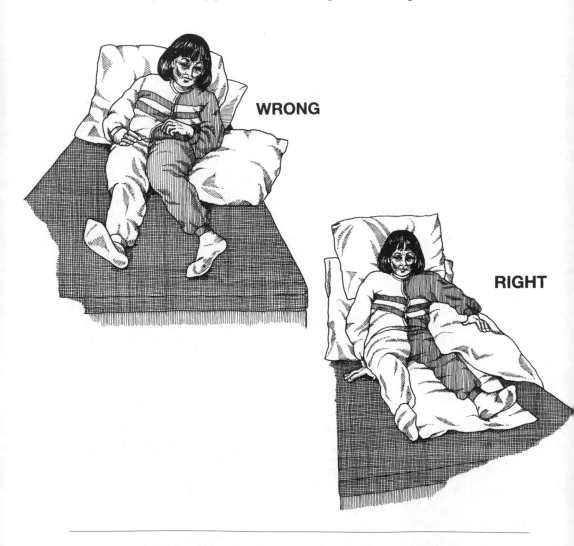

**WRONG**

**RIGHT**

# 5: Getting out of bed

*I think I made his back
feel better.*

Marilyn Monroe, after a private meeting
with John F. Kennedy 1926–62

Once the patient has managed to sit up safely in bed, the next step is to proceed, without delay, to get out of it. Again, the principle of working across the weak side should be encouraged so that the patient gets out of bed on the paralysed side. Pre-stroke, we are in the habit of getting up without even thinking about what is involved. After stroke, most of us will have to break down this activity into a series of movements: rolling over, swinging the legs over the edge of the bed and then sitting up, in preparation for standing.

The correct way to get out of bed after stroke is illustrated in a series of easy-to-follow steps, each of which is shown on the following two pages. *It looks easy and it is!* Are you ready to start?

## If getting up alone your patient should:

1) Bend both knees, using the unaffected leg to help move the weak leg *(step 1).*
2) Roll over onto the weak side.
3) Drop both legs over the edge of the bed. Again, using the unaffected leg to move the weak one, if necessary *(step 2).*
4) Place the unaffected hand on the mattress at shoulder level beside the weak shoulder, and push the body upright *(step 3).*

THE BOTTOM LINE

# The first step in rehabilitation is to get out of bed.

## *If getting up with your assistance the patient should:*

1) Roll over onto the weak side *(step 1)*. You should stand on the side your patient is moving towards and put your hands on the sound hip and shoulder to help the patient roll over onto the weak side *(step 2)*. Help to bring the feet over the edge of the bed *(step 3)*.

2) In order to sit up, put the unaffected hand on the mattress at shoulder level in front of the weak arm. Lift the head and push through the unaffected hand and arm. You can assist by putting one arm on the patient's back between the shoulder blades, and your other arm on the unaffected hip or thigh *(step 4)*.

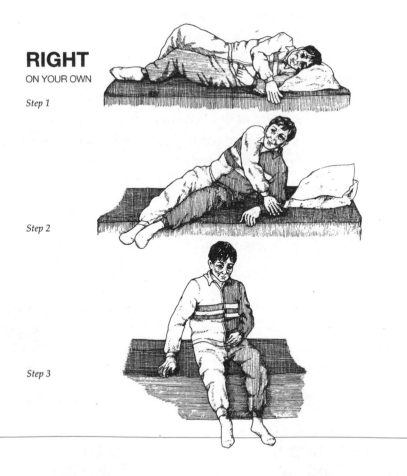

**RIGHT**
ON YOUR OWN

Step 1

Step 2

Step 3

**Carer, please note:**

Do not be tempted to put your hand under the patient's neck. This will not help the movement and may hurt the neck. Also, avoid pulling on the weak arm because this can make the shoulder extremely sore.

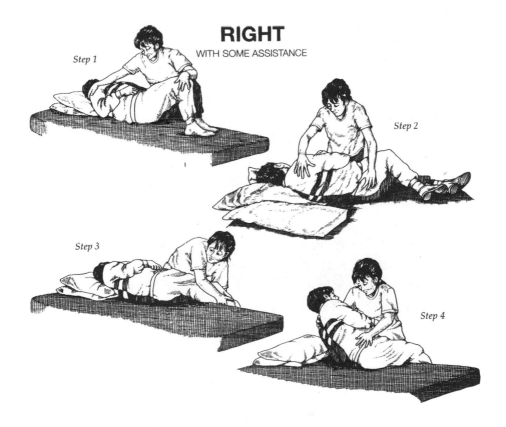

**RIGHT**

WITH SOME ASSISTANCE

*Step 1*

*Step 2*

*Step 3*

*Step 4*

# 6: Standing

*In my view, stability
is a sexy thing.*
Tony Blair 1953–

The next three sections *(pages 112–118)* are addressed primarily to the patient as they contain advice which is best directed at the person who has suffered the stroke. Even if you are not well enough to walk just yet, it can make a refreshing change to see other people at eye level, rather than having to look up from a bed. Try to gradually build up to standing for 20 minutes or more at a time, but don't become disheartened if all that you can manage is two or three minutes at first. Things will improve with practice. They always do, no matter how unlikely that seems at the beginning!

Standing, after being laid-up in bed for a while, is a magnificent way to stretch out the muscles in your legs and back, but you must balance your weight evenly. Do not make the mistake of taking the strain exclusively on the unaffected leg. If you do that the muscles on the weaker side will not be stretched, as indeed they must be for you to become fit and well.

Many of us, when standing for the first time after stroke, may initially need something solid and stable to help steady us: a dining table or a chest of drawers will suffice. It is best to have this positioned directly in front, rather than to the side. You can then rest both hands on the surface and try to distribute your weight evenly before standing upright. In the unlikely event that standing should increase the momentum or frequency of spasm, then do not carry on without seeking further advice from a doctor or chartered physiotherapist.

The correct way to rise unaided from the edge of a bed or a chair is shown

**THE BOTTOM LINE**

Try standing with your carer's arm around your waist.

below. Should you need assistance, the illustrations on the next page will show your carer how to help you.

## On your own

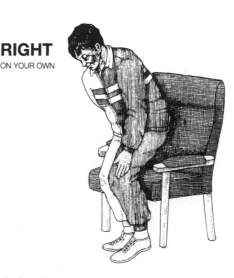

**RIGHT**
ON YOUR OWN

1) Make sure you are sitting on the edge of the bed (or the chair). Your feet should be level with each other and flat on the floor about hip distance apart, tucked slightly under you.

2) Lean well forward so that your shoulders come over your knees and toes. Your feet should be pulled back. Take the weight evenly on both feet. Leave your hands free by your side or push yourself up from the bed (or the arms of the chair if applicable).

3) Rise from the bed or seat and straighten into a standing position.

4) Make sure you are upright, with your hips and knees straight and your weight balanced.

## With some assistance

1) Sit on the edge of the bed or the seat with your feet level with each other and flat on the floor about hip distance apart, tucked slightly under you. Your assistant's legs should be against your weak knee and foot, to keep them in position.

2) Put your unaffected hand on the assistant's shoulder or waist. The assistant's hands go around your waist or hips. Your weak arm should hang by your side, or hold your assistant's waist (if you have enough control).

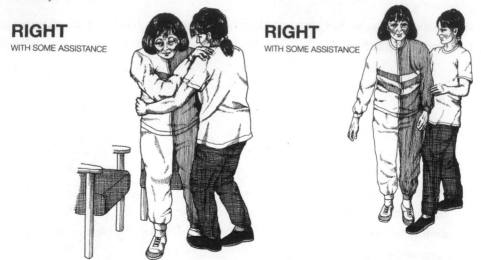

**RIGHT**
WITH SOME ASSISTANCE

**RIGHT**
WITH SOME ASSISTANCE

3)  Lean well forward and stand up. Your assistant helps to bring your weight forward onto your feet and steadies your weak side. Once you are on your feet, you may initially prefer your assistant to continue holding you steady for a little while longer. Just until you become confident enough to stand alone.

# 7: Walking

> ### The business of life is to go forward.
> Samuel Johnson 1709–84

Many people find it difficult to walk initially after stroke. You may find it is hard to take weight on your weak leg or you may fear that it will give way underneath you. To begin with, walk with a wall close to the weak side, in case you should need to prop yourself up against it. Corridors are ideal for this and

**THE BOTTOM LINE**

## To begin with, walk with a wall close to the weak side.

corridors are not hard to find inside hospitals. In some cases, skilled guidance in a physiotherapy department or rehabilitation unit will be necessary. Ideally this should follow immediately after several days of successful standing and sitting practice. Carers, don't be coy in chasing your regional health department or the management of your local hospital trust if this is needed but not forthcoming.

Don't give up, even if you cannot walk as fast as you would like. Try to use your weak side, as many patients find that the more they use the weak side, the less they limp and the faster they can walk. The ultimate goal should be complete naturalness in walking, but this will often take time and persistence. Any limp or dip should be scrutinized and professionally investigated and, if possible, eliminated. The object, as clearly stated by Dr R.M. Youngson in his excellent book, *STROKE!*, is not simply to drag oneself around somehow on two feet, but to do so in such a manner that no casual observer would suspect there had ever been paralysis. It is possible. I and countless others are walking proof of that.

You will find walking easier if you wear low-heeled shoes which give plenty of support. At home, make sure you cannot trip on obstacles such as loose carpets and rugs, discarded children's toys or trailing electric flexes. Also, take care that there is enough light for you to see exactly where you are stepping.

It is most important that you keep practising your walking skills. Otherwise, you may lose confidence. Aim to take a walk each day, even if it is only along a corridor, or down the garden path. You may want someone to accompany you at first. Don't worry if the exertion makes you a little breathless. You will gradually find that you can go further with greater ease.

Two out of three patients find that initially they need a walking aid, usually a walking stick, to help them get around for a while after their strokes. This can help to take weight through the weak side, giving extra support and confidence. If you decide to use a walking stick, it should be at the level of your wrist when you are standing straight with your hand at your side. If it is the

wrong height, it can upset your balance. The stick should be held in your unaffected hand and moved forward as you step forward with your weak leg. A
stick with a crook handle is easier to use than one with a knob handle.

If your foot drops when you step forward with your weak leg and the front
of your shoes scuff the ground, you may find that boots which come over the
ankle, or an ankle splint, can help. Better still, a chartered physiotherapist may
be able to show you exercises to correct the 'foot-drop'.

# 8: Relaxing safely in a chair

### *It was such a lovely day I thought it was a pity to get up.*
Somerset Maugham 1875–1965

In this section, we are going to learn to rest in such a way that our recovery is
enhanced. When relaxing safely in a chair, it's reassuring to know that you can
accelerate your own recovery simply by adopting the *correct* method of sitting
featured on the next right-hand page. Remember, it is easiest to keep your
balance in a chair which has arms and a high, straight back. Be sure to avoid
the *wrong* way of sitting illustrated opposite.

## Sitting down on your own

- Make sure the seat is behind you and that your feet are level and close to
  the chair.
- Reach for the arms of the chair with both hands if you can. If not, reach
  with your unaffected arm (taking care not to lean too heavily on that side).

THE BOTTOM LINE

# Always keep the two sides of the body in balance.

- Lean forwards and bend your hips and knees as you lower yourself onto the seat. Do not flop backwards as you could lose control of the movement and tip over. Take care that you do not sit on your weak hand or trap it against the chair.
- Push your bottom right to the back of the seat.

## Sitting correctly in a chair

When sitting in a chair, some stroke patients tend to slide forward or lean over to the weak side of their body. You may need to correct your sitting position frequently, particularly if your balance is not yet back to normal.

1) Sit in an upright position, with your bottom to the back of the chair and your weight evenly distributed over both buttocks.

**WRONG**

**RIGHT**

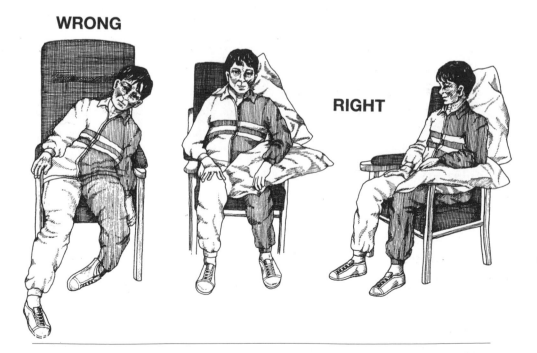

2) Keep your head straight, *not* pulled over to one side.
3) Your hips, knees and ankles should be bent at right angles with both your feet flat on the floor. This is both the correct position *and* the most comfortable way to sit.
4) If your weak foot is not flat on the floor, spasm can develop in your leg which may push it out in front of you and make you slide forward in the chair. Make sure your foot is drawn back to avoid this happening.
5) Your weak arm should be forward and resting on the arm of the chair or on a supportive surface such as a table. A pillow under this arm will give some padding and help to keep it in that position. The pillow should be placed lengthways, tucked into your side and under your weak shoulder.

# 9: Eating difficulties

*The noblest of all dogs is the hot-dog; it feeds the hand that bites it.*

Laurence J. Peter 1919–90

First, I am going to describe the conventional means of dealing with eating difficulties after stroke, then I am going to share with you my way of overcoming the problem. Note that I have no financial interest in the well-known company I shall name.

Eating difficulties after stroke occur for a number of reasons. The most obvious problem is the malfunction of one arm, often necessitating one-handed eating. Many patients cannot manage to manipulate cutlery: pressing the thumb and forefinger together to maintain grip is frequently impossible.

THE BOTTOM LINE

Re-establish your eating skill – one chip at a time?

During the lengthy rehabilitation process the patient may have to use one or more of the following:

- A ROCKER KNIFE. This is a specially-designed knife to stabilize food as it is cut.
- AN OLD-FASHIONED KNIFE WITH A LARGE SQUARE WOOD-EN HANDLE. Much easier for the disabled to grip and control.
- A PLATE GUARD. This device clips directly onto the edge of a plate providing a solid wall against which the patient's spoon or fork can trap food to be scooped up.

Problems of half-vision (*addressed on page 77*) can result in only half the food on the plate being consumed by some patients who have a tendency to ignore everything on their blind side. The solution in the short-term is simply for the carer to turn the plate around halfway through the meal.

Paralysis of the facial muscles and loss of sensation on one side of the face can cause the patient to unknowingly 'pocket' food in the depths of the affected cheek. Fortunately, in most cases, this problem tends to sort itself out in the days following stroke.

In my early days I staggered into a McDonald's restaurant and propped myself up against the counter. When asked, 'What can I get you, sir', I attempted to order but nothing intelligible would come out of my mouth. Undeterred, I just kept on waving at the illuminated menu ahead until the assistant figured out that three shakes of my head and a grunt meant that I wanted the number six burger meal. What followed significantly brought forward my recovery.

Having eaten the burger with my unaffected hand, I began experimenting with mouth and finger co-ordination until I succeeded in aiming *one single featherweight chip* through the gap between my quivering lips exclusively with my stroke hand. After that (to the delight of a bunch of kids who thought my

THE BOTTOM LINE

# Hang on to your sense of humour. You'll be needing it.

antics were for their amusement only) there was no stopping me. I pains-takingly manoeuvred one chip on top of another and, several collisions with my face later, I succeeded in doing *two at a time,* scoring **direct hits onto my tongue!** (While convenience foods have their place, bear in mind that they can be high in salt and unsaturated fat and should only be eaten occasionally.)

# 10: Swallowing

*We will either find a way
or make one.*
Hannibal 247–182 BC

The majority of stroke patients will experience some early difficulties with swallowing. As with many of the undesirable after-effects of stroke, things usually get better over a period. In the meantime, what is needed is a degree of wariness and a few words of advice as follows:

*   Bear in mind that the problem, oddly enough, can be worse with liquids than with solids.
*   Don't hesitate in seeking early advice from a doctor, nurse or dietician.
*   Water, even if some of it goes down the wrong way, is the safest, but not the easiest, fluid to swallow. Sit up as straight as possible, take tiny sips and plenty of time. If it won't go down at all, don't persist. Seek medical assistance if there is any question of dehydration.
*   Sucking a jelly cube is another way to reintroduce liquids but check that the patient can suck.
*   The easiest texture to swallow is a thick, smooth liquid. Soups and some

THE BOTTOM LINE

The easiest texture to swallow is a thick, smooth liquid.

baby foods are ideal for the crucial first few difficult days after stroke. Be sure to avoid foods with 'bits' in, like vegetable soup.

- After eating, check that no food is left in the mouth, particularly down in the well of the cheek on the stroke side where you may have little or no sensation or feeling.

- As time goes by and it becomes easier to swallow, gradually include more and more of your favourite foods so that eating becomes a pleasure once again.

- Do not, under any circumstances, eat too much. The last thing you want to be is an overweight stroke patient because your carer may have difficulty assisting you and the risk of another stroke will be significantly greater.

## *Dribbling*

This comparatively innocent little misdemeanour caused me so much embarrassment and misery. Not only during and after meals, but when socializing up to a year after my strokes and on the pillow at night (that's dribbling on the pillow – not socializing!). One of my least favourite barmen has been known to announce in public, 'You're dribbling again, David'.

The problem is caused by weakened facial muscles. What happens is that saliva pools in the well of the cheek on the stroke side but the patient can't feel it is there. In order to reduce leakage and gradually get the problem under control, here are a few tips:

- Get into the habit of swallowing regularly.
- Always keep a handkerchief or a supply of tissues handy.
- Don't bend your head forward in public – you're asking for it!

# 11: Communication disorders

*He speaks to me as if I were*
*a public meeting.*

Queen Victoria, on Gladstone 1819–1901

Have you ever wondered what it must be like to be sentenced to a period of solitary confinement? Losing the power to communicate comes pretty close. The vital thing for carers and visitors to remember is that stroke patients can still think, feel and hear. They are as intellectually aware as they were before stroke. The difference is that they don't look it, they can't demonstrate it and, most cruel of all, they can't necessarily communicate this all-important fact to you. No matter how much they desperately want to.

Therapists, in addition to their specialized knowledge and skills, are trained to be encouraging, diligent and persistent in their handling of stroke patients. Over time, speech and language therapy can overcome many seemingly impossible disorders of communication.

Carers should try to bear in mind that even the most straightforward and simple tasks can seem enormously testing to the patient. For instance, although I was capable of *seeing* and *thinking* the numbers zero to nine after my two strokes, my accuracy rating for weeks to come was virtually nil. I would see the numeral 4, think 7 and struggle to pronounce 9 (or some other equally irrational sequence). Throughout this period I was adamant that my command of numbers was spot on!

I eventually made slow but gradual progress only when an extremely patient and diplomatic friend took me time and time again through my own telephone number in *numerals, fingers (mine first, then hers), written words and spoken numbers*. Eventually, we graduated to the use of all four routines in the

**THE BOTTOM LINE**

# Disruption is common but generally short-lived.

same visit – one after the other. This discipline proved to be a decisive break-through for me because I caught myself red-handed scrawling the figure *2* on paper and then triumphantly holding up *4* fingers. The almost unthinkable occurred to me right then and there. I was wrong?

My ability with words and numbers and all other areas of communication improved with regular daily practice and careful scrutiny after that. Un-beknown to me at the time, what was actually happening inside my head was that my brain was recovering lost numeracy skills through finding alternative pathways around the stroke-damaged regions.

My friend, who had no previous experience of stroke or therapy, was thrilled to discover that she had been instrumental in substantially aiding my recovery. By trial and error, I discovered that the best time to improve my abi-lity to comprehend words and numerals was immediately after breakfast, before the doctors arrived for their morning round of the wards. At that time of day I would be refreshed from a sound night's sleep and better able to con-centrate, before fading, exhausted, by mid-morning. In the sections that follow we shall further discuss communication disorders and how to set about putting them right.

# 12: Slurring of speech (dysarthria)

*He talked with more claret*
*than clarity.*

Susan Ertz 1894–1985

Healthy human beings communicate with each other in many different ways, including speech, music, body language, gestures, the written word and pictures.

**THE BOTTOM LINE**

This condition is usually temporary.
Get plenty of rest.

When we wish to converse with someone else, it is necessary to put our thoughts into words. This involves the use of language which is essentially a form of coding. If we should discover a bomb under the bed we would quickly need to find a way to warn any occupants of the imminent danger. The image of a bomb exploding in front of our eyes is put into code with immediate effect and the word that escapes our lips is 'BOMB!'

---

### The language sequence

Utterance of the word 'bomb', or any other word you may care to mention, requires the following complex process of planning, co-ordination and execution to take place:

1) The brain will need to work out exactly how to make the appropriate sound.
2) Breathing may need to be adjusted to accommodate that sound.
3) The voice box (larynx) will have to go to work and produce the sound.
4) Muscles in the throat and mouth must get moving to deliver the sound.
5) The tongue, lips, cheeks and nose will need to interact in such a way that the pronunciation of the spoken word is correct

---

Slurring of speech occurs because muscles in the mouth and throat which control speech have been adversely affected and weakened by stroke. Patients sound as if they are drunk, and words frequently come out distorted and unintelligible. Speech deteriorates further when the patient becomes tired or irritated. There may also be some short-term problems with swallowing, chewing or breathing because these actions are controlled by the same muscles.

The important thing to remember for carers and visitors is that there is no need to raise your voice or slow down your own pace of speech. Unless there are other complications, the patient with dysarthria can read, write and understand perfectly well. The only speech-related problem is one of weak muscles in the throat and mouth which should strengthen with time. Most patients recover their powers of speech naturally within a few weeks or months.

# 13: Inability to speak (aphasia)

*Human speech is like a cracked kettle on which we tap crude rhythms for bears to dance to, while we long to make music that will melt the stars.*

Gustave Flaubert 1821–80

To help us understand aphasia (or dysphasia, as it is sometimes called) and to concentrate our minds on the subject, let us return to the bomb under the bed. Patients suffering from aphasia have lost some or all of their ability to decipher language and express themselves in words. This can be one of the most awful losses to cope with after stroke.

## Ideas can no longer be converted into the correct words

Depending on the severity of aphasia, patients may not speak at all or they may use incorrect words. In many cases errors bear some resemblance to the intended word. For instance, a bomb may be called a boom, a bop, a rom.

**THE BOTTOM LINE**

Speech therapy is the answer. Success will take time.

Furthermore, errors in speech tend to be inconsistent. The patient may refer correctly to the bomb one day, but call it a womb, the next.

Understandably, those patients suffering from aphasia, like the rest of us, try to appear as normal as possible. They may respond positively to an invitation to have a cup of tea, but gentle probing may reveal that even the words 'yes' and 'no' are used inappropriately. The patient has lost the ability to encode and decode language. It can seem as if everyone, including loved ones, is speaking a foreign language in which the patient is not fluent.

## *Aphasia causes loss or impairment of the ability to use language accurately*

Deficits include:

- Inability to find the correct word.
- Use of nonsensical sayings.
- Difficulty in understanding what other people say.
- Awkwardness in grouping words together in a sentence.
- Impairment of speech, reading and writing.

With this condition, the services of a highly-trained and experienced speech therapist can often be crucial to recovery. Thankfully, I have no personal experience of severe aphasia to offer you. In my opinion, the most moving and inspirational account of a woman's comeback from this predicament is recounted in the autobiography of Barbara Newborn, *Return to Ithaca*, published in the UK, USA and Australia by Element in 1997.

# 14: Caring for an aphasic person

*Let thy speech be short,*
*comprehending much in*
*few words.*
Ecclesiasticus 32:8

You know how frustrating it is to misplace a word, to have it on the tip of your tongue but not be able to bring it to mind. For the stroke patient with aphasia (who already has many other deficits to contend with) it feels like that all the time. The battle for words can be soul-destroying. Not surprisingly, the patient can get angry, frustrated and tearful.

Carers should speak in a simple, straightforward manner, using easy to understand language. Too much should not be delivered in one mouthful as many aphasic people are easily confused by complexity.

Ample time should be allowed for ideas to be assimilated. Every channel of communication must be explored. Carers should always try to supplement their facial expression by gestures or by other helpful means. If the written word is more easily understood than speech, or if writing proves to be an aid to comprehension, then this should be used to communicate, no matter how slow or tedious this may seem. All that really matters in the end is that the patient recovers and you both feel good. How long that takes is of secondary importance.

In the early weeks following stroke, a spontaneous phase of recovery normally occurs in all but the most severe cases. After a few weeks or months, the pace of recovery slows and things can get difficult. Proper motivation and a meaningful purpose in life, albeit a long-term goal, are essential in promoting optimum recovery at this stage.

## THE BOTTOM LINE

# Some way of communicating **must** be established.

Stroke patients and their carers already have a potent cocktail of problems to contend with. The disturbance of the language function alone is enough to try anyone's patience. Speech and communication with others are central to our most basic human needs. Except in certain rare cases of stroke where extensive brain damage has led to an abnormal lightening of the patient's mood, some degree of depression is an almost universal feature in the early months of an aphasic patient.

Regardless of the ups and downs of rehabilitation and recovery (and in my experience recovery can go on happening for years), do not lose sight of one essential truth: depression, no matter how frightening, does not last forever.

# 15: Speech and language therapy

*Conversation has a kind of charm about it, an insinuating and insidious something that elicits secrets from us just like love or liquor.*

Seneca 4 BC – AD 65

A competent and dedicated speech therapist can provide tremendous help, motivation and support. The relationship between patient and therapist is all-important. Life being what it is, it is unrealistic to expect two strangers to immediately feel comfortable and relaxed with each other on first meeting. It helps if the patient can demonstrate their willingness to work and co-operate. The therapist can be relied upon to do a professional job.

### THE BOTTOM LINE

## Most stroke patients recover their speech in the end.

## *A speech and language therapist can help by:*

- Diagnosing precisely what is wrong.
- Explaining how things can be improved.
- Advising patient and carer on new and innovative ways of communicating.
- Making the relearning process stimulating and enjoyable.
- Contacting the appropriate local voluntary support groups.
- Monitoring the patient's progress.

## *The carer can assist at home by bearing in mind the following*

We all perk up and concentrate when our interest is aroused, but most of us have diverse and different interests. If a football fanatic is trying to read, the write-up of yesterday's big match is the obvious text. If a woman loves her garden but is unable to manage the practical side just yet, encourage her to sit outside and have fun touching, smelling the aromas and naming the plants and flowers, which can be stimulating if not always accurate.

Anything which brings stimulation and excitement into the day is a bonus. If the atmosphere is alive and sparky there will be extra alertness, increased concentration, heightened awareness and a major boost along the way to ultimate recovery. Number one in the stimulation department is laughter, more laughter, and even more laughter still. Then there is companionship. This is the moment when friends can really demonstrate their worth. I think I learned, for the first time in my life, what friendship is all about when I was really ill.

### An extract from Barbara Newborn's autobiography

For the first six months, I found myself breaking apart, shifting, desperately searching for new answers. In the hospital, as I looked around me, I began to realise that faith, support and laughter might be the qualities that matter most, making life worth living again. The smiling faces around me seemed remarkable. I was not the only one with tragic problems. Everyone there seemed to sense what pain and illness were. Some patients were helping each other, silently reinforcing the message, "*You are not alone.*"

# 16: Occupational therapy

*The greatness of human actions is measured by the extent to which they inspire others.*

Louis Pasteur 1822–95

Contrary to popular belief, the role of an occupational therapist (OT) is not to find you a new occupation, but to help you gain as much independence in life as possible, particularly with essential daily living activities. These professionals tend to be very much in demand and invariably in short supply, so if you are allocated one, either in hospital or at home, make the best of your good fortune.

Patients who were not admitted to hospital after their stroke, or their carers, should consult their doctor or local social services department who will put them in touch with an occupational therapist or home care assistant should the need arise.

**THE BOTTOM LINE**

## Occupational therapists help you to help yourself.

Their first priority is to help with basic things like washing, dressing, toilet routine, personal care and the preparation of food and beverages. The art of occupational therapy is to teach and cajole their charges into doing everything for themselves that is within their capability.

Recovering from stroke and adapting to temporary incapacity or lasting disabilities can be a long and soul-destroying process, particularly for the elderly and the severely disabled. Occupational therapists know only too well that the patient's psychological outlook can greatly influence progress in adapting to their handicaps. They are trained in basic motivation and morale boosting techniques. Where necessary, they will arrange for special equipment to be installed in the home, or for adaptations to be made to the home, prior to the patient's discharge from hospital.

Despite the millions of strokes that occur worldwide every year, no two strokes are identical. Everyone who has a stroke is affected in disparate ways. The one universal feature of successful stroke recovery is the individual patient's will to get well. That alone, in some cases, can make the difference between total independence one day and a wheelchair for life.

Occupational therapists and home care assistants have a major part to play in the rehabilitation of stroke patients. It will be, as always, the exclusive domain of the patient to decide if they want to make the enormous effort required to regain their independence. If, and only if, they do, the occupational therapist's dedication and hard work will eventually result in a better quality of life for that patient.

# 17: Fast-track ways to get better

*I believe the only way to get*
*ahead is just to get on with it*
*and learn from one's mistakes.*
Richard Branson 1950–

Most stroke patients are not only keen, they're downright anxious to be as independent as their incapacity will allow. Others are not. It is essential to be caring and helpful towards the disabled but too much kindness can be counterproductive. If patients are given help unnecessarily they will expect it again and again. Soon, they will become accustomed to dependence and may feel disinclined to struggle. Efforts towards self-help cease.

When help is needed (with dressing, for example), it is better to assist only with those parts of the operation that the patient finds troublesome than to perform the whole task. As skills improve, patients should be left to get on with more and more, so that they gradually become increasingly independent.

The first few days after stroke are none too soon to begin trying to win back faculties impaired by stroke. Small pleasures, activities which are stimulating but not too testing, will count for much and boost morale and motivation no end. My bed in the clinic where I was convalescing after discharge from hospital was situated on the ground floor, adjacent to the fire exit. Naturally, at times when I felt stronger (usually following a lengthy snooze), I couldn't resist the temptation to break out and take a few steps onto the warm August lawns to the rear of the establishment. I would lie down under the sun, on the grass, in my striped pyjamas.

I was discharged one Saturday morning and spent the next 24 hours in bed, recovering from the upheaval of being transferred from one side of town

**THE BOTTOM LINE**

# Establish a routine to regain handgrip and foot control.

to the other. On waking the following morning, I resolved that today, and every day for as long as it took, I would wage war on my physical disabilities. I knew, from sad experience in hospital, that I wouldn't be able to comprehend my usual Sunday newspaper, but I was, nonetheless, going to make it round to the nearby newsagent and get one. I was determined to make myself carry it back with my stroke hand. Any offers of help would be refused.

The round trip of a few hundred yards took forever. I propped myself up against walls and sat down to rest on doorsteps until eventually I made it. I couldn't lift the quality papers; they were too heavy. After shaking out all the enclosures (easy, my hand was shuddering so much, the little leaflets jumped out of their own accord!) I made off with a tabloid on the basis that it was the lightest in terms of weight.

I dropped it 27 times on the way back. I had difficulty manipulating my hand and the wretched thing would repeatedly judder itself out of my grasp. No matter; I gathered all the crumpled sheets together again and continued. By the time I got back, my prize was reduced to pulp and I was ready for bed. *Yet I was winning.*

# 18: Driving

*Everything is possible. Faith is
the substance of our hopes...*
Henry Ford 1863–1947

After stroke, never allow yourself to forget there is an exciting and real world beyond your own doorstep. Subject to your doctor's advice and the practicalities of your particular circumstances, it will usually aid your convalescence to get out there and enjoy it as much as your limitations will allow.

**THE BOTTOM LINE**

## Get back in the driving seat as soon as you're fit.

Even in the 21st century, driving is still a pleasurable activity for most people because it gives us independence and the ability to get out and about at will. In the majority of cases, driving ability will be impaired by stroke in the short-term, but most patients find that they are able to return to the driving seat within a few months.

There are, however, two stroke-related conditions that expressly preclude driving. One is epilepsy, which affects around five per cent of stroke patients. The other is a major disturbance of vision. The most common visual impairment after stroke is half-vision, an inability to see on one side *(see page 77)*.

Driving restrictions vary from country to country. In the United Kingdom, for example, anyone who has experienced a stroke must not drive for at least 30 days after the event. Both the licensing authority (the DVLA in the UK) and the driver's insurance company must be informed. As soon as clinical recovery is satisfactory and your doctor gives you the go ahead, driving may be resumed. If there is a residual limb disability, a restricted licence may need to be issued limiting driving to vehicles with controls suitable for the relevant disability.

The sensible thing to do, when getting back behind the wheel after a period of absence from driving as a result of stroke, is to go out with a qualified driving instructor, preferably one with a knowledge of stroke.

If you are fortunate enough to have a choice of cars, a two-door saloon allows easier access to the front seat than a four-door model. An automatic vehicle is simpler to drive than a manual car, but you may need professional tuition before switching from one to the other.

In the event that you are a newly-disabled passenger being transported by car, the best seat for you is the front passenger seat. See if you can move the seat as far back as possible by yourself and recline it slightly. Ask for assistance if necessary. This will allow you maximum room for manoeuvre.

*Avoid the use of a disabled parking permit wherever possible.* Many disabled people, of course, have a genuine need, but even in the days when I was deemed to be disabled, I would rather struggle than admit that I was incapable of walking 100 yards from a public car park to a doctor's surgery. Even in my worst times, after my second stroke, I have only ever been prepared to admit to temporary incapacity, never disability. Why? I was afraid it might become a permanent reality. After all, it does not take long to create a habit.

# 19: Counselling

*After my initial consultation I was positive I'd made the right decision. I was made to feel at ease, that there was nothing to be ashamed of.*
*The relaxation exercises and therapy have greatly helped. They allow me to keep situations in perspective and remain calm. They bring peace of mind. It's comforting to know there is someone working constructively with me to overcome this setback.*
Mrs S.F.

Ill health – our own, or that of a loved one – often generates uncertainty, worry, fear and distress. It can lead to high levels of stress. We may lie awake at night worrying about our health, our partner, money, incapacity or what the kids are up to. Sometimes these concerns become more diffuse and turn into

## THE BOTTOM LINE

There is boldness, not shame, in seeking help.

general feelings of anxiety. At this stage, panic, which is an extreme form of fear, can begin to overwhelm us.

Too much anxiety may ultimately result in a panic attack. To avoid this unnecessary complication in the aftermath of stroke, the heat must be taken out of a stressful situation before panic breaks out. Counselling, which involves providing the stressed person with tangible strategies and techniques in order for them to come to terms with their anxieties, can work wonders for both stroke patients and carers. It can help by getting to the root cause of psychological problems and addressing them. All of those butterflies in the stomach can, with therapy, be made to fly in the same direction!

## A competent and qualified counsellor can assist in the following ways:

- **Listening in a professional and relaxed manner.** This alone has been shown to be one of the most significant factors in helping people minimize the negative effects of stress.
- **Identifying primary objectives.** This is often necessary because we do not always stop to ask ourselves what it is we really want from life. In my case, as you would expect from a former stress counsellor, I was very clear in my mind exactly what I wanted: complete recovery and back on my feet and going somewhere by the year 2000.
- **Assertiveness training.** Assertion is a much misunderstood word. It is not about getting your own way all the time. It is about being straightforward and rational in your relationships with others and also involves having respect for yourself and other people. Being self-confident is the basis of assertion. Understandably, this is not easy for stroke patients to master, but it is possible.
- **Encouraging natural response skills.** Quite simply, this is the reassurance necessary for stroke patients and others to produce an appropriate

response to situations. For example, when you are sad, you cry; when you are happy, you laugh. It is a fact of life that both tears and laughter have a therapeutic effect.

- **Relaxation techniques,** some of which we touched upon on pages 31–34. Relaxation reduces muscular tension and gradually empties the mind of stressful thoughts.

- **Hypnosis and hypnotherapy.** Some medical practitioners, psychologists and a number of stress counsellors are additionally qualified in the art of hypnosis. This procedure can be beneficial in trauma removal and in the negating of deep-rooted fears and inhibitions.

# 20: Dance therapy

*Do not take life too seriously.*
*You will never get out of it*
*alive.*
Elbert Hubbard 1859–1915

It doesn't really matter whether or not you can dance. The most important thing in your world is to succeed in making the best possible recovery from stroke available to you. Dance therapy has a role to play in helping to accelerate that recovery. Lack of a convenient or willing dancing partner, if that is the case, is of little significance. Indeed the inability to get out of the house doesn't prohibit you from enjoying it either. Providing you have reached the stage of being stable on your feet (with or without a walking stick) this therapy is a must for you. Persevere, if only for a few minutes each day and you will feel better, get better, and maybe have some fun!

**THE BOTTOM LINE**

To enjoy oneself is the expressway to recovery.

Some people can succumb to the view that because stroke is such a serious setback, one should be sombre and sad forever more. This attitude is wrong and to some extent accounts for the abysmal degree of recovery that many patients record, despite the clinical fact that the majority should have the capacity to get better.

Fellow strokers, it's not a sin to have fun and enjoy your recovery. Push the boundaries of your physical and mental deficits to the limit, then rest. I know it's tough, but for the sake of your future quality of life it has to be worth any effort. Dancing has proved to be therapeutic for me, even in the days when I have been unable or unwilling to go out.

Apart from eating breakfast, there are two things I do, every weekday morning, before settling down to work. One is described in detail on page 156, the other is dancing my way through the household chores. Yes, I grab hold of a duster or the upright vacuum cleaner, whatever takes my fancy, put on some music to bop to and dance all around the flat.

My taste in music to get me mobile varies. At the present time, I only have to hear the sound of *Mysterious Times* by Sash, or *Killin' Time* by Tina Cousins, and I'm instantly swinging, even when standing still. After three or four repeats, I'm ready to tap along with Michael Flatley, the vacuum cleaner, or anyone foolish enough to visit me before noon.

---

### Try it!

Others might think you are mad, but then you and I have been to hell and back and survived. We know best!

---

# 21: Pathways to happiness

*...I'll build a stairway to paradise*
*with a new step ev'ry day!*
*I'm going to get there at any price;*
*stand aside, I'm on my way!*

George Gershwin, Arthur Francis, Buddy Desylva

With a positive attitude of mind, a degree of competence and a 'can do' approach wherever possible, you can achieve fulfilment and happiness in life. Life after stroke can indeed be tremendously rewarding, but first you have to tackle the tricky bit. You must struggle to turn misfortune around and put it to work for you. If you think of yourself as a victim, **STOP!** Don't permit yourself the luxury of labelling yourself with such a convenient and negative cop-out.

You have probably read many books on positive thinking and perhaps you agree with the technique, as indeed I do. But be careful. Positive thinking, no matter how positive your attitude of mind, will achieve nothing on its own. For positive thinking to lead successfully to fulfilment and happiness, we must find and incorporate the other essential ingredients. Just as flour without water and a hot oven will not make bread, positive thinking without a degree of competence and a 'can do' approach to life will lead nowhere.

In the days when I used to run a commercial training organization, I saw thousands of people – including some of my own staff – who refused to think and act with any degree of competence. They wanted everything to be easy and instantaneous and to fall effortlessly into their laps. They are the people who always were, and, sadly, always will be, (unless they change their ways) disappointed in their hopes for fulfilment and ultimate happiness.

**THE BOTTOM LINE**

Oh yes you can! You **can** be happy again someday.

I did not ask to be struck down by two strokes but without this misfortune I would never have bothered to restructure my life. There is an element of making a virtue out of necessity but, I believe that these days, I am stronger in character and spirit and significantly more humane as a result of my clash with fate. I was damned if I would roll over for a couple of strokes and you too can benefit from this difficult phase in your life if you consider your future health and happiness to be worth fighting for.

Whenever I read a book that I am determined to benefit from, I devour it. I read each line again and again if necessary until I have fully grasped the meaning of every word, marking with a yellow highlighter the passages that strike me as being of crucial importance.

To gain maximum benefit from this book, to create a truly satisfying lifestyle for yourself following your recovery to come, you must do the same. Devour this book, extract all the information that could be useful to you, then set about putting the essential principles and tips you have learned into *action*.

Recovery may not be easy, instantaneous and swift. Three years elapsed before I felt almost completely better, but what is three years in an entire life-time? **Nothing less than an opportunity to learn how to be happy.**

# PART SEVEN

# depression

# 1: Stroke and depression

*You have no idea what a poor
opinion I have of myself – and
how little I deserve it.*

W.S. Gilbert 1836–1911

The tragedy of depression, which affects more than one in ten otherwise healthy adults at some time in their lives, plus a formidable fifty per cent of stroke patients, is that it can creep up slowly and envelop the patient in a thickening black cloud of energy-sucking misery, extinguishing almost all of the joys of living. Women are more prone to depression, but men are more difficult to diagnose because they find it difficult to ask for help and frequently disguise their mental and emotional symptoms as physical problems.

The number of people affected by depression is rising fast. Recent figures from the World Health Organisation suggest that depression will become the second-biggest health problem in the world by the year 2004. It is distressingly common in stroke patients who remain, to a large extent, in possession of their mental faculties but who have difficulty speaking or communicating in other ways.

Patients with a past history of depression, together with those who were of a gloomy and pessimistic disposition before their stroke, are more likely to be affected. But, quite frequently, depression can take hold of a previously cheerful and active individual who now has to contend with the frustrations and restrictions that accompany incapacity or disability.

Very often, stroke patients who are depressed are easily distracted as well. No matter how intelligent the individual, it can be difficult to concentrate on even the most simple of tasks at times. There's a certain debilitating heaviness

**THE BOTTOM LINE**

# Depression, although frightening, is never permanent.

to depression that seems to the afflicted to accentuate the force of gravity.

I am no stranger to depression. In my teens I was hospitalized for 10 weeks with clinical depression. Throughout my life, approximately once every seven to ten years, I've had to go into battle mode to evict that devious, invisible lodger from my mind. In the 1980s and early 1990s, when I used to treat clients suffering from depression in my own stress management consultancy, I thought the problem was history in respect of myself. How wrong could I be? Nothing on earth could have prepared me for the absolute depths of depression to which I would sink in the aftermath of stroke. Not directly afterwards, but increasingly during the 28 months that followed.

Don't be alarmed. I can laugh about it now. Whatever happens to you on the way ahead, always remember this one absolute truth: **depression, although frightening, is never permanent.**

# 2: The downward spiral of depression

*In the real dark night of the soul it is always three o'clock in the morning.*

F. Scott Fitzgerald 1896–1940

For the first time, *the bottom line* below is neither practical nor inspirational, it's defeatist. Why? The depressed person knows. But the patient's family and loved ones, unless they have suffered the misery of depression themselves, cannot understand why their well-meaning and genuine attempts to give comfort and help are ineffectual. In the next section *(pages 145–146)*, I am going to give you just one brief glimpse of the terrifying isolation in which severely

**THE BOTTOM LINE**

## The motivation to help oneself is simply not there.

depressed stroke patients can find themselves trapped, based on my own personal experience.

My uncomfortable slide down the spiral of depression, after successfully overcoming many of the challenging and incapacitating aspects of stroke, might, in this enlightened age when most forms of depression are now treatable, have been avoided altogether. Like many men (women are more sensible about consulting their doctors on emotional matters) I was not prepared to admit that I just couldn't cope.

Another disincentive for me to seek help from my doctor (and perhaps for those accustomed to the previous generation of antidepressants like Valium), was that I had spent much of the 1980s and early 1990s weaning over-stressed clients off such drugs so that they could reclaim their real selves. In those days there was no non-addictive wonder drug that was safe to use. One that really worked. There is now! We shall discuss Prozac on pages 147–148.

Nearly all of us feel miserable and depressed at some time or other, perhaps when a love affair ends or when redundancy is looming. But for many stroke patients who have already suffered brain damage and who must adapt to a completely different way of life, depression is not merely a passing phase. It can cause apathy, loss of interest, a pessimistic view of everything, uncontrollable floods of tears, insomnia and a depth of sadness that only those afflicted would recognize. The effect of depression can be so devastating that, for many, the only escape they can visualize in the absolute depths of depression is suicide.

Like stroke, each experience of depression is unique and different. The patient feels alone and helpless in a personal nightmare way beyond the reach of family and friends. One of the most distressing aspects of the condition and, perhaps, the reason why depression is so difficult for family and friends to understand, is the feeling of isolation in which the patient seems trapped.

# 3: 'Black dog'

*...And now my life has changed*
*in oh so many ways;*
*my independence seems to vanish*
*in the haze.*
*But every now and then I feel so*
*insecure,*
*I know that I just need you like*
*I've never done before.*

Lennon & McCartney

Samuel Johnson, known as Dr Johnson, coined the phrase 'black dog', when referring to his attacks of melancholia in a letter to Mrs Thrale in 1783. More recently, Winston Churchill used the phrase when alluding to his own bouts of depression. Here in the third millennium, depression is about as common as a family with a dog and, as an illness, it does have a certain animal-like ferocity about it. One that is not keen to let go once it has you in its grip.

The condition can be unpredictable, however, relaxing from time to time to give you respite – a moment, a day, a week or maybe more to pick yourself up – but you know from bitter experience that it has not done with you yet. It has not really gone away; it's merely lurking, out of sight, ready to pounce when you least expect it. Do you cry for help? Do you tell your friends? Of course not! Like me, you are too ashamed. You do what you think will be best for everyone, you shut yourself away. Then, before you know it, the beast is back with a vengeance! Do you care? Not any longer, things have become altogether much too unbearable to care. You are consumed with despair, isolated and desperate.

**THE BOTTOM LINE**

I **cannot** help myself just now.

Then the telephone rings. You answer on impulse, trying hard to sound normal and in control, but the caller asks how you are and that touches a raw nerve. Try as you do, you just can't fake it, you burst into uncontrollable floods of tears and put down the phone, physically and emotionally exhausted. You are ill, you are suffering from depression.

Surprisingly, I allowed myself to become ill with depression after doing so well in my endeavours to recover from stroke. I became increasingly withdrawn and would seldom venture outside. And things got worse, far worse! My niece, Jane, alerted by distress calls from neighbours and the community warden, would try to gain access to my flat.

She banged and banged on the front door for so long I had no option but to answer it. I wrenched open the door and glowered at her. If looks could kill she would have been a goner. She politely asked if I was all right. I said, 'No,' and shut the door in her face.

By the following Sunday, I felt so awful something made me press the autodial for Jane at work. She answered straight away, but I was too emotionally out of control to say anything but her name. By coincidence, my sister, who would normally have been at home 200 miles away, was with her. They were both round within minutes and they were shocked. Nothing could have prepared my sister for the inconsolable wreck that she encountered on arrival. Jane had already had a glimpse before.

That day, although unpleasant for all three of us, was a watershed. It cleared the way for a new beginning. Neither of them, however willing, could have helped me until I was ready. But on that one occasion when I was not only ready, but receptive, they were there.

# 4: Prozac

*You see things; and you say,*
*'Why?' But I dream things that*
*never were; and I say, 'Why not?'*

George Bernard Shaw 1856–1950

Prozac has become the most popular anti-depressant in the world. The manufacturers claim that patients typically show an improvement in their condition two to three weeks after being prescribed the drug. Unlike previous generations of anti-depressants which were highly addictive, Prozac is not addictive and has fewer undesirable side-effects. The active ingredient in the drug is fluoxetine and this inhibits the re-uptake of the brain chemical, serotonin, boosting chemical levels in the brain and maintaining the brain in a higher state of arousal (not depressed).

It works!

Prozac has acquired a reputation for helping patients overcome not only their basic symptoms of depression, but also a range of other problems which, until recently, were traditionally thought to require psychotherapy or counselling. Such problems have included a lack of self-esteem, fear of rejection and extreme sensitivity to criticism, issues that can frequently manifest themselves in the minds of patients as a direct result of stroke. The drug is often prescribed for elderly stroke patients with depressive symptoms because older patients are considered to be able to tolerate the same starting dosage as younger patients.

**THE BOTTOM LINE**

## If all else fails consult your doctor about Prozac.

## Coming off Prozac

Many previously depressed people swear that Prozac has been their salvation and some, who are no longer depressed, continue to use it to help their social life go with a swing. Understandably, since it doesn't appear to do users any harm and the side-effects can be relatively mild, these people may be in no hurry to discontinue its use and many will stay on the drug indefinitely. Psychiatrists, I suspect, and indeed, friends of mine who are psychologists, do not approve of the notion that anti-depressants should be used to improve one's personality.

## Will I suffer withdrawal symptoms?

Suddenly discontinuing any form of anti-depressant treatment can have serious consequences for a minority of users although Prozac is less likely than other drugs in this group to cause problems because it is metabolized very slowly in the human body. Choose the ideal time to gradually scale down your dosage as a preliminary to withdrawing from the drug altogether. A period when something exciting is happening in your life is the perfect time to quit. At the very least, ensure that things are moving your way and you have definite and absorbing interests in life.

If you are, or can be, physically active during the duration of your withdrawal, so much the better. Even in the unlikely event that you 'land heavily' and experience the flu-like symptoms caused by too-rapid cessation of the drug, all is not lost. You simply return to full dosage for a short period, then, by arrangement with your doctor, you progressively scale down your dosage to zero over time.

# 5: A purpose in life

*Take time to deliberate, but when the time for action has arrived, STOP THINKING AND JUMP IN.*

Napoleon Bonaparte 1769–1821

So…this is your dilemma…Although you are now considerably better than you were in the days immediately after your stroke, you are nowhere near as able as you would wish, and you are not at all sure that you will ever be happy again.

Furthermore, you're fed up, frustrated and bored and you would dearly love to have something interesting and rewarding to do. And, if that's not enough to contend with, you're getting older by the day and you shudder to think what the future holds for you. You're grateful for the help and care you've received, of course, but you just won't be happy until you have something worthwhile to occupy your time.

'Is that too much to expect?' you may well ask.

'No, it is not,' I would most certainly reply.

The following is a true story. The evidence is still hanging in my hallway at home.

I was passing the local community centre (formerly the village school) when I noticed there was a local art exhibition taking place. I spent a leisurely hour browsing through the various paintings on display before selecting a colourful picture of five children flying a kite. It wasn't the technical merit that attracted me to it, it was the similarities to an old-fashioned birthday card my Aunt Freda, crippled from birth and born with no neck, once painted for me as a child.

**THE BOTTOM LINE**

## Rediscover, or find, a purpose for your life.

I noticed that the picture was simply signed 'Lois' and, when handing over the money at the cash desk, I enquired if the artist was from Polperro. 'She lives in Looe, five miles along the coast,' I was told. 'You've only just missed her. She was here a few minutes ago. She's 90, you know, and not so well these days. I can't wait to tell her we've sold her painting. It will make her so happy.'

If you feel a rumbling discontent with your life, stop reading for a moment and consider realistically what would make you happy. Do you have a meaningful purpose in life? If not, you have the most wonderful discovery ahead of you when you find it or perhaps rediscover it. Since recovering from stroke illness, I no longer have the inclination for the cut and thrust of business or the desire to resume my former profession, although both gave me tremendous satisfaction at the time. Some while back, when I was last in hospital, I found myself reminiscing about my younger days and all those things I had wanted to do, but never done, such as writing the type of books that I believe to be worthwhile.

Decide on your purpose in life. Would by the time you finish this book or soon after be a reasonable target? Nothing will keep you more alive and it can also be the foundation of your future happiness.

# 6: Death of a loved one

*The sound of her silk skirt has stopped.*
*On the marble pavement dust grows.*
*Her empty room is cold and still.*
*Fallen leaves are piled against the doors.*
*Longing for that lovely lady...*
*How can I bring my aching heart to rest?*

Han Wu Di, Emperor of China,
on the death of his mistress. 156–86 BC

*Life is a great surprise. I do not*
*see why death should not be an*
*even greater one.*

No one lives forever. Sometimes we have to face the painful reality of the patient we have cared for dying and leaving us all alone. In the United States and Britain alone, almost 10 million people every year experience the death of a member of their immediate family. Personally, when I lose someone very special to me, I derive much comfort from the quotation above by Vladimir Nabokov (1899–1977), author of *Lolita* and *Pale Fire*.

Grieving over the death of a loved one is a natural way to release emotional feelings and our traditional way of making peace with whoever has been taken away from us. The process takes time and cannot be rushed. Many people choose solitude as their way of coming to terms with what has happened. For others, equally devastated by their loss, the comfort of others is what they need. For most of us, grief is punctuated with periodic bouts of tears.

**THE BOTTOM LINE**

## Allow time to grieve in your own special way.

Sooner or later, there comes a time to let go. Touch can be instrumental in opening up the pathways to emotion and help to release the anguish of grief. When we are trying to hold back painful emotions, we clench our muscles, locking in memories and thoughts that we have difficulty in dealing with. The professional touch of a masseur or a masseuse, in a relaxed and private environment, can have the effect of allowing blocked emotions to flow more freely. It is possible that you may shed some tears during therapy so it is a good idea to mention your bereavement when phoning for an appointment. Don't just book for a 30-minute session; book for the whole hour.

Or perhaps you would consider bereavement counselling from which many people have gained much solace?

The change of seasons can provide a change of focus and a turning point in your life. Even in the death of winter we can see snowdrops rising from beneath the snow. If you have access to a small piece of soil and a few seeds, why not plant a miniature garden of remembrance? Many people find that growing new life in mourning soaks up some of the pain associated with bereavement.

# 7: Pet therapy

*If what you want is cuddling,*
*you should buy a puppy*
*(or maybe a little kitten).*

Julie Burchill 1960–

Animals have an important role in society as therapists. Marjorie Unwin, who is in her 60s and spent two months in hospital recovering from stroke, was featured in *Stroke News* in 1998. She said, 'My swans give me a reason to get up

**THE BOTTOM LINE**

# If the nature of your depression is loneliness, get a pet.

every morning. I'm lucky to have them to live for. I was shown photos of them while I was in hospital. They are my life so I had to fight back. They got me better.'

Directly en route from my flat to the village of Polperro lies a picturesque snow-white bungalow set back from the road on a hill, overlooking the river. Whenever I walk past the property, young Linus, a lovable King Charles spaniel, will 'yap' excitedly and come bounding across the lawn to greet me at the garden gate.

His owner, Carmen, is blind, but that doesn't stop her walking into the village most days to shop and enjoy a chat with her friends. She gets there and back safely enough. Linus sees to that! More than that, he pays his way by keeping Carmen on schedule every day. When it's breakfast time and Linus is feeling a bit peckish, Carmen tells me he will come bounding into her bedroom, jump up onto the bed and give her lots of licks and kisses, until she gets up and feeds him.

On cold winter days when Carmen might not otherwise bother to pop out for some fresh air, Linus is the one that can make all the difference. He knows perfectly well that if he can prompt her into action and lead her down to the Old Mill House tavern, not only will he get his regular ration of dog biscuits from Joe, the cellarman, he will be able to laze in front of a blazing log fire. If Carmen is not well or if there's a problem (no doggy food by sundown, for example), Linus will simply bark at the garden gate until a passing local comes to investigate.

Esmond Gay, a former patient who suffered a nervous breakdown, attributes his recovery to the happiness he has derived from breeding rare Bengal cats.

Why not consider a pet for yourself or your patient? The comfort and unconditional love provided by a warm, furry creature is often the precursor to being able to feel human love again as well.

# 8: Quality sleep

*A man can only do what he can do. But if he does that each day he can sleep at night and do it again the next day.*

Albert Schweitzer 1875–1965

While we sleep, essential self-maintenance and repair work is taking place throughout our bodies. Physical changes are taking place at the same time. For instance, blood pressure drops and both breathing and heart rate slow down. In the months following my second stroke, when I was partially paralysed on my right side, I would always try, despite pain or discomfort, to position myself in bed in the pre-stroke position. I figured that if I could force my body to rest for the night in the correct position, it might regain the habit of normal posture. The strategy seemed to work, but it is a very slow process best started just as soon as you are physically able.

How did I achieve this? By persistent trial and error and by flatly refusing to accept that I would make anything less than a complete recovery. Every time my arm or hand or both adopted the limp *paralysed* position while I was still awake, I would use my unaffected hand to gently reposition my stroke side to imitate a normal position.

I remember waging war with my right foot in 1995. For the last three weeks of August and September in its entirety, my foot wanted to drag and flop. I wanted it to perform like a normal foot and I was in no doubt that I had the moral right to consider myself boss in this matter. Every night in bed, using my unaffected foot alternatively as a prod and lever, I would gently manoeuvre it into a respectable position before dropping off to sleep. In the end, I think

**THE BOTTOM LINE**

## Sleep is the natural watering place for body and soul.

my foot accepted that it was less trouble to perform as required.

All this sounds simple enough but, of course, it requires not only determination, but plenty of rest too in order to be able to continue the self-help therapy in the morning. Stroke patients generally need far more rest than healthy people. They must also strive harder than most to achieve mobility on the affected side of their body. How is it possible to reconcile these conflicting demands?

My solution was to plan every day in advance. If I had something planned for late-afternoon or the evening, I would either get up late that morning, or rise as normal but take a two-hour siesta in the afternoon. To complete this book on schedule, I would work for as long as my brain was willing to function, or until the first warning signs of physical fatigue set in, then sleep for as long as I needed, regardless of what time in the day or night it was.

Before bringing this section to a close, forgive me for stating the obvious, but I once had a friend with a bad back whose bed was literally collapsing beneath her. You spend a third of your life in bed. Doesn't it make sense to invest in a firm, supportive bed? If finance is a problem, sell the car and get a bed. It's that important to your recovery.

# 9: Bath time

*I have had a good many more
uplifting thoughts in well-
equipped American bathrooms
than I have ever had in any
cathedral.*

Edmund Wilson 1895–1972

If I had to point to one single external factor that has facilitated my recovery more than anything else, it would be my bath! No routine, time-saving showers for me. Every day, without fail, complete with aromatherapy oils and herbal essences, I have a heavenly hot bath lasting an absolute minimum of one hour, sometimes two! If the telephone rings, I just leave it to ring. If somebody knocks on the door, I ignore it.

You might consider this to be discourteous to callers. Possibly, but my defence is that I noticed long ago there is therapeutic benefit to be had from a leisurely bath. **It is much easier to manipulate stroke-ravaged limbs in water.** Be warned. Elderly and disabled patients should consult their doctor before putting into practice the suggestions on this page.

'Rub it better' is a phrase that we have all known since childhood. The action of rubbing increases the blood circulation in the damaged area, helping to promote the healing process.

Give yourself a massage the next time you are enjoying a bath. Start by using your unaffected hand to gently massage your stroke side. As you get better, make the effort to use your stroke hand to massage the other side of your body. It doesn't matter that your efforts may be feeble and non-professional to begin with. The mere effort of trying will stimulate your stroke

THE BOTTOM LINE

# Bath time can be supremely therapeutic for you.

arm and hand to some extent and it will also re-establish the fact that your stroke side has a useful role to play in your life.

Have fun! Massage your partner, the dog, or anyone else who happens to be in the bath with you at the time.

Soaking in hot water (or warm, if you prefer) relaxes and soothes both your mind and body. Don't rush it – this is as good as liquid therapy gets! If your facial muscles have got themselves all in a tizzy over stroke this is a good time to gently massage the contours of your face and mouth. Position a mirror where you can see it from the bath and practise smiling. Don't worry about cracking the mirror with your early attempts to smile, your facial muscles will become increasingly taut with regular practice and you may eventually be pleased with the result.

# 10: Aromatherapy and massage

*If you want a thing well done, get*
*a couple of old broads to do it.*
Bette Davis 1908–89

Men, forget all about the steamy massage joints of Bangkok. We are talking here about highly-respectable practitioners in aromatherapy and massage, based principally at hairdressing salons or beauty parlours, but also accessible through the phone directory.

Men, why am I singling you out for special treatment here? The therapeutic benefits of aromatherapy and massage have played a major part in my recovery from stroke and depression. Even now, I go for regular sessions because I have no intention of slipping backwards. How is it, that whenever

**THE BOTTOM LINE**

Experience the healing qualities of scent and touch.

and wherever I go, all the other clients are invariably women? Could it be that most males are too petrified to phone for an appointment?

Massage releases tension, frees energy, removes physical blocks and feels good. It also brings awareness to the sensory nerves – just what you need after stroke – and can increase circulation, ease pain and provide passive exercise. Always insist on a qualified and experienced aromatherapist. Give your therapist full details of your stroke.

## The healing benefits of plants (aromatherapy)

As we smell an aroma and breathe, the essence is picked up by the hairs that line the nose, and traces of the essence travel through our olfactory system on nerve impulses directly to the brain. At the same time, our lungs draw in tiny molecules of the plant essence mixed together with oxygen. One whiff of fresh lavender, for instance, can reduce anxiety and tension by altering our physiological responses. Essential oils have a variety of properties that are helpful to stroke patients and individuals suffering from depression: my personal recommendations are the calming and relaxing properties of sandalwood, tea tree, bergamot, lavender, geranium, camomile and ylang-ylang. Take care when handling essential oils and never apply them neat to the skin. Readers who wish to use the oils themselves would be well advised to read up on the subject first. An ideal book for beginners is *Principles of Aromatherapy* by Cathy Hopkins (Thorsons).

## The age-old therapeutic benefit of massage

Massage has been shown to reduce blood pressure, alleviate some types of headache, and has been used effectively in the treatment of depression brought on by trauma. A study at the University of Miami Medical School in 1993 demonstrated that depressed patients who received the benefit of a half-hour massage had consistently lower levels of stress hormones during the massage and afterwards. Patients also reported they were able to sleep better.

One of the great joys of massage is that you are helpless on the couch with nothing to do. You have little choice but to lay back and let your therapist do with you as she will. Just allow your body to go limp and try to empty your mind of all thoughts. If you find yourself thinking or worrying about anything, simply abandon your thoughts for the time being and revert to the unparalleled luxury of lying there and being pampered in the name of therapy.

# 11: High anxiety

*Nothing in the affairs of men*
*is worthy of great anxiety.*
Plato 427–347 BC

If you want to be happy in life, keep all your commitments, but don't expect other people to keep theirs. When making a commitment, however small, we give our word. Giving something as valuable and as powerful as our word is not to be taken lightly. When we are prevented from keeping our word, quite apart from disappointing others, we subconsciously begin to mistrust ourselves to a degree. Over time, the accumulated effect of countless broken pledges extracts from us a heavy penalty. We reach a stage in life when we begin to have serious self-doubts. A general feeling of being ill at ease takes hold.

Self-doubt has a tendency to feed our perception of unworthiness, causing tiredness, confusion, lack of clarity and a mounting sensation of high anxiety.

## THE BOTTOM LINE

Anxiety is fear spread thin and wide like a pizza.

Some people live their lives in a constant state of anxiety. They wonder why they can no longer enjoy even the most basic pleasures in life. What, you might wonder, has this to do with *me*?

Your best chance of recovering from stroke is to clear your diary of all commitments so that you can concentrate exclusively on getting well. Let others know (if they need telling) that it's self-help for them while you give your all to regaining your precious faculties.

You have already made a substantial investment in renewing your health in a number of directions, not least by reading this book. You may have been capable of doing many things at once in the past. You will probably do so yet again in the future, but just now, after stroke, there's only one priority – getting better.

## Typical causes of high anxiety

- SERIOUS ILLNESS. A major stroke inevitably comes into this category.
- CHANGE. An unexpected upheaval in lifestyle, although stressful at the time, can be beneficial in the long-term, as I have discovered to my great delight.
- YOURSELF. The exasperation of coping with yourself in a brain-damaged state, or the responsibility of coping with a loved one ravaged by stroke, would surely test the best of us. You may emerge a stronger personality as a result of your brush with adversity.
- OTHER PEOPLE. You may be filled with alarm at the thought of others viewing you as someone who is incapacitated and disenfranchised. I know I was.
- LACK OF COMMUNICATION. Carer – imagine what it feels like to be a stroke patient who has something to say, but cannot speak. Those who care must find some means of communication, albeit by touch, eye contact, graphics, written words, nods or, ideally, a combination of all these.

- TOO MANY DEMANDS. The very next section was written especially for you!
- WORRIES, SELF-DOUBT AND BROKEN PROMISES. The next but one section on page 163 is going to throw you a lifeline: the chance of a whole new beginning.

# 12: Defusing anxiety bombs

*Write to amuse? What an appalling*
*  suggestion!*
*I write to make people anxious and*
*  miserable*
*and to worsen their indigestion.*

Wendy Cope, author of *Serious Concerns*
1945–

The last thing you want in your life, after the trauma of stroke, or during a period when you have the added responsibility of caring for someone in need, is unnecessary anxiety. If you are the patient, you will be aware that your brain has been damaged by stroke. Providing you have the capacity to recover, you can learn to cope adequately again in time because all human brains come complete with back-up capabilities to deal with most types of stroke emergency. Nevertheless, you are bound to feel confused, frustrated and downright defeated at times. The chances are that you will be hit by an anxiety bomb unless you learn to disarm the trigger of tension before it overloads and fires from within.

## THE BOTTOM LINE

# Much anxiety you can simply choose to do without.

## My way

In the very same year that I had my two strokes (1995), I instructed both estate agent and solicitor, from the comfort of my hospital bed, to sell my oversized and redundant house. I relieved myself of all remaining responsibilities, large and small, by simply putting my company into voluntary liquidation. In another form, in other hands, it lives on to this day, continuing with the work of counselling clients with anxiety related problems.

You could say I was fortunate that my second wife had already divorced me, and my girlfriend left when the going got tough because this left me free and unencumbered to concentrate on the business of getting well. Others (the vast majority of readers, I suspect) might argue that it is infinitely better to have your partner at your side in times of need. No matter. Providing the patient learns to disarm any potential trigger of tension, it is possible to cope in either of these circumstances.

## How to disarm the trigger of tension and relax

It's easy, but you must stick unwaveringly to the two essential rules that conclude the next section *(page164)*. Don't be deceived by their simplicity. They work! All you have to do to defuse potential anxiety bombs in your life is adopt the anxiety block that follows on the page opposite. You will then be in a position to concentrate exclusively on the only thing that really matters to someone who has lost their health: **getting better!**

# 13: Anxiety blocking

MACBETH: *Canst thou not minister to*
*a mind diseased,*
*Pluck from the memory a rooted sorrow,*
*Raze out the written troubles of the brain,*
*And with some sweet oblivious antidote*
*Cleanse the stuffed bosom of that perilous*
*stuff*
*Which weighs upon the heart?*
DOCTOR: *Therein the patient must*
*minister to himself.*
Shakespeare 1564–1616

---

### THE ANXIETY BLOCK

'I am feeling fitter and happier. Physically, I will begin to feel stronger and more able. I will get more confidence, and because of this feeling of confidence – *which I can feel in my very fingertips* – I will be able to face things more easily. I feel this confidence welling up inside me, and I feel rested and calm.

'Every day, in every way, I feel better and better. I find it easier to concentrate, and as I do concentrate, I feel a deep sense of security, comfort and happiness. I find that my thoughts are less centred upon myself, and as each day goes past, I feel stronger in my mind and in my body.

'INNER PEACE are my key words for instant calm.'

---

**THE BOTTOM LINE**

# INNER PEACE are my key words for instant calm.

## The rules

- CLEAR OUT THE UNNECESSARY CLUTTER FROM YOUR LIFE. Start today. If you are too ill to reason or act, you should have someone trustworthy to perform this function for you.
- READ ALOUD, OR SILENTLY TO YOURSELF, THE WORDS OF THE UNIVERSAL ANXIETY BLOCK ON THE PREVIOUS PAGE. Say it profoundly, with deep-seated passion, three times a day until you are completely well, or until such time when you have realized the best possible recovery available to you. Sit or lie down before you commence this powerful ritual. Always remember to take three slow, deep breaths before you begin. Never forget.

# 14: Break out!

*I am ready for Fortune
as she wills.*
Dante 1265–1321

Who knows what will do it for you? A chance encounter, a fascinating new interest, a real challenge, or perhaps it will be a book or a renewed sense of purpose that causes the gloom to lift. For some it will be the undying love of their partner or a new friendship that will banish the blues in the end, or an unexpected act of kindness from a distant relative, or simply one single ray of light.

Remember, depression, however frightening, is never permanent.

Many patients experience that wonderful day when darkness and despondency inexplicably fade away. Some may put this apparent miracle down to a

**THE BOTTOM LINE**

Up the spiral you come. Welcome back to the world!

change in the weather or sheer good fortune. Others, including myself, can look back with clarity to a definite turning point. In my case, it was the help of a friend who was struggling to combat cancer for the second time in her life. I wrote the opening pages of this book whilst cat-sitting in her house as she lay on the operating table in hospital. There were muddy brown paw prints all over the first draft of Chapter 1. You've done pretty well yourself, haven't you? You have survived a crash course in depression (not everyone's choice of an ideal read!) and I wager you could manage a smile?

## *Learn to play again*

Maybe we should learn to play again. When I've finished this book, I'm seriously thinking of buying myself the best train set money can buy. My friends will laugh at me, of course, but do I care?

When did you last observe young children at play? Kids can be disarmingly therapeutic and uplifting to watch because they have so few inhibitions. In the days when I used to counsel highly-stressed clients from my consultancy at home, my three-year-old daughter, Danielle, would delight in asking any clients who were waiting in the lounge to draw her a cat! With her oriental eyes wide with expectation, she manoeuvred her sketch pad and pen onto their defenceless lap, smiled enchantingly and waited. She never failed to elicit a cat! Sadly, despite her ice-breaking skills with the clients, I had to call a halt to her little games. She had somehow figured out that it was Daddy's job to make the visitors feel better. One day, I came into the lounge to hear her enquiring, arms crossed and immovable in front of the client, 'So, what's the matter with you, then?'

Phone a friend and arrange to meet. Do something (legal) totally out of character just for the hell of it. Get some excitement back into your life! Book a holiday or at least a weekend away. Go to church or throw a party. Pick up the pieces and start living again.

# PART EIGHT

# adjustment

# 1:  Drama and tears

> *In spite of illness, in spite of sorrow, one can remain alive long past the usual date of disintegration if one is unafraid of change, interested in big things, and happy in small ways.*
>
> Edith Wharton 1862–1937

At some inopportune moment after stroke, you will become aware that you are a more sensitive person than you were before. This discovery, which may well be accompanied by tears, could result from a domestic crisis, no matter how minor, or simply from the act of watching television. Stroke has impacted disproportionately, as it always does, on your feelings and emotions. At times during rehabilitation, your mood – indeed, your entire frame of mind – can be affected by trivialities. This, thankfully, is but a passing phase, albeit a difficult one. It can be traumatic for some people, particularly men, to find themselves suddenly and uncharacteristically prone to fits of uncontrollable weeping, especially when it happens in public.

For almost two years after I was released from hospital, I could barely bring myself to watch anything but comedy on television. I was incapable of watching The News without being overcome by melancholy at the very first item of tragic, or even moderately bad news. Drama on the screen, let alone in real life, seemed to affect me a hundred times more than before.

Stroke patients will eventually succeed in getting their emotions back

**THE BOTTOM LINE**

Avoid upsetting drama or news on TV.
Opt for comedy.

under control, but it can take a very long time indeed. I knew I was fine, three years later, when I felt confident enough to go to the pictures again with a friend. I made it almost to the end of *Titanic* without the need to hide behind my giant carton of popcorn.

This increased degree of sensitiveness is not all bad news. After a trying three years, adjusting to the new me, I find that I am a more considerate person than before.

Carers should bear in mind that patients must be encouraged to reconcile themselves to their changed personality and adjust to different circumstances, otherwise recovery can never be complete. Try not to tolerate any unreasonable demands or behaviour. You may succeed only in slowing down the desired recovery and making your own life arduous and increasingly unhappy into the bargain. Too much help and kindness can have precisely the wrong effect.

If your patient is not prepared to struggle and endeavour to get well, whatever the odds, then your time is better served as motivator, not facilitator. And that involves being firm when necessary. Don't allow your own life to become unbearable. Apart from your duty of care to your patient or loved one, you are most certainly entitled to a life too. A good and meaningful one.

# 2: Facing the future

*Life is like playing a violin
in public and learning the
instrument as one goes on.*
Samuel Butler 1835–1902

Stroke is not only devastating for both patient and carer, but also for family and friends because it has the potential to dramatically change the person they know and love. Caring for someone after stroke can be difficult and stressful. After the initial trauma, many carers understandably go through feelings of loss and grief for the lifestyle they used to enjoy. It is not unusual to experience feelings of anger, resentment, guilt, inadequacy, anxiety or depression because of the responsibilities of fulfilling a role for which one has not been professionally trained.

Experienced carers suggest that you:

- Share your feelings with someone (another carer, perhaps) who understands what you are going through.
- Get information about support services and assistance available in your area (refer to the resource directory at the back of this book).
- Accept as much help with the daily routine as possible.
- Make absolutely sure that you take regular breaks in order to recharge your batteries.
- Keep in touch with your friends and have a good laugh whenever possible. *Remember, laughter is potent medicine not only for patients, but for hardworking angels too.*

**THE BOTTOM LINE**

We, stroke patients and carers, possess hidden talents.

## *The good news*

Caring for someone with stroke illness is not all bad news. Far from it. My family has been drawn closer together by the trials and tribulations I have encountered. They, along with some of my closest friends, derive well-deserved satisfaction from my recovery. They know, even though they may have been driven to distraction at times, they are the ones who made a difference: their individual contributions mattered.

I would like now to tell you about someone whose tragedy was far greater than mine, someone whose courage and determination to get well was so remarkable that she created a novel way of improving her stroke-damaged body. Not only did Margaret Humfrey succeed in helping herself but, in partnership with a friend, Pippa Bartolotti, she established a thriving garment business.

When Margie was 21 she suffered a massive stroke. After 32 years of constant difficulty and struggle, she developed a weighted body band that helped to gently coax and nudge dormant muscles back into activity and fitness. It did wonders for her sense of co-ordination, balance, mobility and confidence. In recent years these highly-effective weighted body garments and bands, which are worn under everyday clothing, have been made available to other stroke sufferers and the long-term disabled. (For details, see the resources section at the end of the book.)

# 3: Self-determination

*Real greatness consists of*
*being master of yourself.*
Daniel Defoe 1660–1731

I was greatly moved by Barbara Newborn's story of her triumph over the disabilities of stroke. In her engaging self-help book, *Return to Ithaca* (Element), she puts forward the enlightened view that there are no good and bad experiences in life; what makes life good or bad is what we do during and after our experiences.

Barbara was a 22-year-old student teacher in America when she experienced a severe stroke. The experience of stroke was bleak and disillusioning, she writes, but on the other side, there was an oasis waiting where she uncovered more joy and compassion than she had ever known. 'The healing starts when you allow it to begin,' she says, at the end of her book.

I wholeheartedly agree with those words of wisdom, born of her own experience of stroke. The first step to self-determination and recovery has to come exclusively from you. Notwithstanding the limited control you have over your surroundings and prospects, despite the restraints on movement imposed by incapacity or disability, with all due deference to your advancing years, IT IS STILL POSSIBLE TO BE MASTER OF YOURSELF, TO SHAPE YOUR OWN DESTINY AND TO ENJOY THE YEARS REMAINING TO YOU.

Understandably, with all the confusion and mayhem that has been going on in your life since stroke, your confidence and self-esteem will have taken a tremendous pounding and you may have lost your way. Now is the time to focus on your inner strengths, not deficits, and to let go of the past. **Let's draw a line under the past once and for all.**

### THE BOTTOM LINE

# The healing starts when you allow it to begin.

## Allow the healing process to begin

Today, should you decide to make it so, could be the definitive turning point in your life, the all-important moment of self-determination. Stroke has created, however inconveniently, the opportunity for a new and unexpected adventure in your life. Seize it! Think about what you would most enjoy doing with your new life, *that one thing that excites you and unleashes the most creative forces from within.*

Don't allow your thoughts to be restricted just because you can see no immediate prospect of making things happen. You never know how circumstances in the coming months and years may move in your favour. To my surprise and amazement, they certainly did for me, likewise for Barbara Newborn and countless others. Why not for you?

Often, the experience of stroke, compounded by life in general, has deadened both patients and carers alike to that special spark within them that can ignite the potential for fulfilment. Give yourself a real chance of self-determination, open your mind and let your thoughts dwell for a while on what would make you really happy. Allow the healing process to begin.

# 4: Increasing self-confidence

*The key to greater self-confidence is birth control:* **control** *over the birth of your own* **thoughts!** *Abort all* **negative** *thoughts about yourself, nurture only* **positive** *thoughts.*

An extract from the LCI Practitioner Training Manual (Volume 1), 'Stress Management, Analysis and Bio-feedback' by David M. Hinds and Jackie Thomson

## Confidence boosting

There are five general physical and psychological activity zones in which confident people engage to improve or maintain their self-image. They are of prime importance after stroke.

1) **Image and attitude:** Accept that your attitude will suffer if you don't maintain a positive self-image. Even if you are not concerned about how others view you, care about how you view and value yourself.

2) **Personal appearance:** Devote time and effort to an exercise programme devised and controlled by a qualified physiotherapist. For the long-term disabled and patients with stroke-damaged bodies, innovative body bands and weighted garments are available via mail order (see resources section).

3) **Letting go of negative habits and traits:** Just imagine how great you would feel if you succeeded in kicking a habit that you have wanted to quit for years. No anti-social habits? How about undesirable character traits? Could there be scope for improvement here?

**THE BOTTOM LINE**

# Think positively about yourself and your recovery

4) **General health:** Are you maintaining a balanced and healthy diet after stroke? Do you have any additional problems that would benefit from a consultation with your doctor? Have you taken your doctor's advice (and any medications prescribed) in respect of all existing conditions? Are you incorporating the necessary lifestyle changes into your daily routine to reduce the possibility of another stroke? Have you come across any suggestions so far in this book that might benefit you? Will you use them?

5) **Simplifying your life and being yourself:** The world around you is becoming increasingly complex. For you, at this moment, it may be beneficial to concentrate on simplicity. Simplify your life and focus on what is important to you and your carer. Dare to be yourself, even if that means being different from other people.

## *Satisfaction can be a great confidence booster!*

The most satisfying way to boost our confidence in ourselves is to *do* something good. What is a good thing? *You* decide. For some people, including those of us who are recovering from stroke, it might be trying out a new or different way of doing something. For others, devouring a book might be just the ticket. You may feel inclined to visit, phone or write to a friend. Or to forgive someone who did you a disservice. It could be something spontaneous, exciting and unexpected: offering someone a helping hand, an encouraging smile, a compliment, or a long-overdue thanks. Again, the key here is **doing**.

# 5: The self-fulfilling expectation

*Nothing extraordinary, great or beautiful is ever accomplished without thinking about it more often and better than others.*

King Louis XIV 1643–1715

Such is the power of the mind that people who expect to lose their memory as they grow old usually do. But loss of mental function is not an inevitable part of ageing. Many people in their 70s, 80s and 90s achieve magnificent feats. Think, for example, of the astronaut, John Glenn, still whizzing around in space almost a generation after most pilots retire. Or Herbert von Karajan, the former conductor of the Berlin Philharmonic Orchestra, performing well into his 80s. The comedian, George Burns, was still active on his 100th birthday!

There is mounting evidence that the self-fulfilling expectation is a factor in determining the degree of recovery or rehabilitation following serious illness. Patients who have the capacity to recover and a positive outlook frequently recover better than those who are pessimistic. What this means is that over time we are liable to become what we think about most; what we expect to happen tends to happen.

Our perceptions determine what we actually experience in a given situation because they make us receptive to some stimuli and blind to others. Those of us who expect to find problems in a given situation are usually able to find them, while those of us who expect to find opportunities in the same situation will also be successful. No two strokes are ever exactly the same but whereas one patient might feel bitter and disinclined to struggle, another, of similar age and deficit, might battle to get better and succeed.

**THE BOTTOM LINE**

## Think about getting better. Always.

Our outlook on life determines what we perceive in a situation and this is particularly relevant when it comes to recovering from illness, or caring for someone who is. Those of us with an optimistic, self-directed outlook somehow expect to find ways of coping, no matter how bad things look at first. Whereas patients or reluctant carers with a pessimistic outlook doubt that they can cope and very often they don't! **Sometimes they don't bother to try.**

How would you characterize your own outlook? Can you discern any persistent patterns in your outlook that may be preventing you from doing your best? For each negative pattern that you identify, create an image of the positive thought form with which you would like to replace it. For example, if you find it difficult to ask for help, think how you feel when someone asks for your help and you give it. You feel good, don't you? At regular intervals, over the next few days, practise holding positive images in your mind. You will be gratified at how much your overall outlook can be changed for the better when you assume the responsibility to control your own thoughts.

---

REMEMBER, OVER TIME, WHAT WE EXPECT TO HAPPEN TENDS TO HAPPEN. **THINK ABOUT GETTING BETTER. ALWAYS.**

# 6: The nursing home option

*And here I still am, unable to do anything for myself. I am nursed day and night, and have to be turned. But there is the television and unlimited reading matter.*

Dirk Bogarde 1920–99

The majority of patients who have been hospitalized by stroke will ultimately be well enough to continue their convalescence at home, usually within a matter of weeks or months. Unfortunately, a small minority, less than 10 per cent of those admitted to hospital with stroke-related deficits, cannot return home. In some cases, this is because their disability is such that going home is no longer an option. In others, usually the frail and very elderly, patients are all alone in the world and understandably too traumatized, or stroke-damaged, or both, to be expected to cope adequately without ongoing care and supervision.

## Residential and nursing home care

A residential home provides personal care and meals in a relaxed and congenial environment while a nursing home provides more intensive support with qualified nurses on the premises. For the majority of people in need, residential and nursing home care is arranged through the local government social services department. The first step is to get a comprehensive and professional assessment of the level of care required. This can be arranged through a hospital social worker for patients already in hospital or by contacting the welfare department or social services direct.

**THE BOTTOM LINE**

## You are not alone.

Whether you are considering residential or nursing home care for your-self, or for someone else, it is worth visiting several homes before making your final choice. For the purposes of researching this page I visited several homes in my area. I found that it was possible to get a general feel for the standard of care and commitment shown to existing residents simply by watching the staff go about their duties. The relaxed and good-humoured smiles, or otherwise, on individual faces speak volumes without a word being spoken. Many homes, usually the better ones, are quite happy to let you chat away informally with the residents.

For the carer charged with the responsibility of finding the right home for a difficult, frightened and probably highly-distressed stroke patient, it is essential to choose a home with previous experience of accommodating the depressed and stroke-damaged. Listen carefully and heed the advice of profes-sional carers|. They know, from extensive past experience of placements, which homes are more suited to your particular charge.

# 7: Independence

> *'You should not bite the hand that*
> *feeds you,' the proverb warns. But*
> *maybe you should, if it prevents*
> *you from feeding yourself.*
>
> Thomas Szasz 1920–

Independence is not based upon physical ability or disability. If at all possible, don't give up activities you enjoy. Adapt them to suit you or seek help to enable you to continue. Whenever, despite your best efforts, you find that it is no

**THE BOTTOM LINE**

## Independence is a state of mind.

longer feasible to carry on with your favourite pursuits, use your time and ingenuity to discover alternatives.

I assure you, from the experience of having my business, my personal ambitions and my private joys dashed by stroke, there is a whole world of happiness out there just waiting for you. But you have to look with enquiring eyes, otherwise opportunity could stare you in the face and you wouldn't see it.

Just because you see other people severely affected and disheartened by stroke, it doesn't follow that you must succumb to a similar state of mind. If you allow yourself to believe that you will never again exercise complete control over your arm and hand then you probably never will. Alternatively, if you can convince yourself, despite current difficulties, that you really want to move your arm and hand again, then you are already one step towards achieving your goal.

The next step is to imagine that you can! Close your eyes and steel yourself to mentally manipulate first your arm, then your hand, and finally the individual fingers of your hand. Slowly and carefully, with extreme concentration, imagine in your mind's eye that you are actually doing it. Over and over again. Next, do it passively. Hold your stroke hand with your unaffected hand and show your stroke hand exactly how the sensation of scratching your leg is accomplished. Demonstrate this procedure to your stroke hand every day with love, conviction and patient persistence, until such time as you feel confident enough to try it for real with your stroke hand.

Don't expect results too soon, but if your preparation has been good and thorough and you are determined to succeed, you might just see a glimmer of movement. This, indeed, will herald the start of your real recovery. Despite the possibility of further disappointments to come, you will go on getting better and better over time. Develop this skill until that magic moment when, all of a sudden, you become aware that your efforts have been rewarded: your muscles are, once again, obeying your commands.

# wellbeing

# 1: Accepting yourself after stroke

*It is the chiefest point of
happiness that a man is
willing to be what he is.*

Desiderius Erasmus 1466–1536

Self-acceptance, confidence and self-esteem come from *doing* things. These sought-after personal qualities come from successfully working around disabilities and obstacles rather than breezing to success with little effort. This is the fundamental reason why patients who are trying their best, regardless of the severity of their stroke, stand an exceptionally good chance, better than most lottery winners, of finding true happiness in the end.

A good example of self-acceptance is Dick Heckstall-Smith, a 65-year-old rhythm-and-blues jazz musician. He accepted his new starting line when two strokes, back in 1992, left him unable to speak, read or write. He could, however, still remember tunes from his childhood and, incredibly, he was able to play his saxophone as well as ever.

A self-confessed eternal optimist, Dick refuses to allow his strokes – or fear of another – to interfere with his career. Here is a quote from an interview with him in *Stroke News* (published by The Stroke Association, Winter 1998 edition):

> Of course I'd rather be alive than dead, so I do take steps to avoid further strokes, such as not smoking and changing my diet. I test my blood pressure every day, but it's always at its lowest just before I go on stage to play. Curious, but true! As for the future? I'm going on tour in Germany and I'm looking forward to recording my next CD with guitarist, Eddie Martin.

**THE BOTTOM LINE**

# Self-acceptance allows you to be at ease with yourself.

Self-acceptance allows you to be comfortable with all aspects of your after-stroke self. You might well be incapacitated or have any number of ongoing disabilities, but you feel confident that you are doing everything in your power to minimize this sad interruption to your life. Because you no longer feel the need to compete with others, you can proceed at your own pace to overcome the various setbacks and difficulties that you have to contend with. You can choose to be yourself; you don't need to fit into the mould of society's out-dated conception of the unhappy typical stroke patient. Stroke management is moving forward in this new millennium. Things are getting better. There are greater opportunities for patients to do worthwhile things.

One of the most rewarding aspects of self-acceptance is that you can at last be at peace with yourself, the good and the bad. Your confidence and self-esteem grow in tandem because you like yourself more. There's no need to build a fortress around yourself, no need to guard against others seeing the real you.

# 2: Zest for life

> *There is more treasure in books*
> *than in all the pirates' loot*
> *on Treasure Island…Best of*
> *all, you can enjoy these riches*
> *every day of your life.*
>
> Walt Disney 1901–66

Allowing for your current limitations, what is it that you really like doing? Whatever it is (unless it's harmful to yourself, or others), DO IT! If, for any reason, that is not possible, put in motion the necessary preparations to make

**THE BOTTOM LINE**

## Reach for your treasure chest!

it become possible within a realistic timescale. If you cannot think of anything on this earth that you would really like to do, then experiment. Try something new. You have nothing to lose and everything to gain by trying.

Be creative. It doesn't matter that initially you might not be too good at it. It doesn't matter if you make mistakes along the way. What does matter is the process of doing which in itself is therapeutic. It can help to put you back in touch with the general flow of life.

The possibilities are endless. A leisurely trip to a bookshop or library will open your eyes to literally hundreds of hobbies, pastimes and sources of income suitable for people recovering from stroke. For those who are completely housebound, access to the Internet is just a few easy-to-learn clicks away with your hand. Here are a few suggestions:

- READING FOR PLEASURE OR EDUCATION. Walt Disney certainly knew how to thrill others and enjoy himself. His every word about the riches to be mined from books on the previous page is spot on. If your eyesight is not what it used to be and an optician cannot help you, sit back, get yourself comfortable and listen to a talking book.
- COMPUTING, WRITING OR ACCESSING THE INTERNET. Until 1997, I had never used a computer and I do empathize with those who are absolutely terrified of the things. Many of the horror stories you may have heard throughout the 1990s were probably true at the time, but these days computer programs really have become user-friendly. Access to the Internet opens up an exciting new world of possibilities for you, including linking up with other stroke patients from around the world.
- JOINING OR HELPING TO ORGANIZE A **LOCAL** STROKE CLUB. The Stroke Association in London and similar organizations around the world can supply you with the specific information you want.
- SKETCHING AND PAINTING. The sheer pleasure, the sense of achievement and the therapeutic benefits of this and other creative pastimes can

be immeasurable. Severe muscle weakness is often a problem and supports are available to compensate for this.

- GARDENING AND OTHER ACTIVITIES. Despite incapacity, many people are at their happiest creating beauty from the soil. With such a vast spectrum of choices available, the odds are in your favour that you will indeed find that special something to interest you.

# 3: Plan for recovery

*There is no failure except*
*in no longer trying.*
Elbert Hubbard 1859–1915

## THE STARTING POINT
## Think it, dream it, plan for recovery and **strive for it.**

Decide now exactly what it is you want out of life! Do you want to milk your role as victim to the full and bathe in unadulterated sympathy? Of course you don't! You wouldn't be reading this self-help book it you were that type. Do you want to try, tough as it is, to piece your life back together again, bit by bit, as best you can? Would you like to benefit from this terrible ordeal and go on to find happiness and satisfaction in life? Good, here's how to do it.

## *Your personal recovery plan*

1) **Focus** exclusively on getting yourself fit and well. You can deal with other matters later.

2) **Be gentle with yourself.** Whenever you have exerted yourself, rest and take it easy for a while directly afterwards.

3) **Choose your helpmates well.** Avoid negative thinkers and patients who have given up on the will to live. They will feed you negativity and drag you down if you let them.

4) **Consult the experts.** In order to secure the best possible recovery available to you, you should now ask your doctor or physiotherapist to assist you in the preparation of your stroke recovery plan. Refer them to this page of the book when asking for their assistance.

5) **One step at a time.** Mountains are climbed, and the seemingly impossible achieved, by taking just one step at a time. That's how your recovery is going to be achieved.

6) **Humour.** Try to see the funny side of efforts to help yourself that misfire! If you can laugh in the face of this catastrophe you will be well insulated against any setbacks you may encounter in the future.

7) **Be flexible.** As your recovery accelerates you'll discover shortcuts that can lead to further progress. At other times you will take one step forwards and two backwards. Press on regardless!

8) **Be willing.** Don't let how you feel about your condition stop you from doing what needs to be done. As soon as you can, physically move your stroke-damaged body in the direction of your ultimate goal. Commit your goal to paper. Write it down at the foot of this page.

9) **Turn fear into excitement.** They both consist of the same basic ingredients, energy and feeling. The only thing that makes them different is your personal interpretation. Change the course of your life today. TURN WON'T POWER INTO WILL POWER!

> MY NAME IS ........................................................................................................................
>
> MY ULTIMATE GOAL IS ........................................................................................
>
> ..................................................................................................................................................

# 4: Working from home

*Much of the world's work, it has been said, is done by folk who do not feel quite well.*

J.K. Galbraith 1908–

Working from home, no matter where in the world you live, can be a source of great pleasure and satisfaction for the elderly, the retired, the recovering stroke patient and the disabled. It would take an entire book to run through all the commercial and voluntary opportunities open to stroke patients who wish to do something useful with their lives. Providing that you have a telephone at home, and you are well enough to use it, you could be in business from your favourite armchair!

If you have a computer, or if you are prepared to acquire one and learn how to use it, access to the Internet is easy and a whole new world of self-employment possibilities open up for you right in front of your eyes. The last time I spent a pleasant few hours surfing the Internet, I came across dozens of

**THE BOTTOM LINE**

If you have a good mind, the opportunities are endless.

opportunities potentially suitable for the enterprising disabled person working from home. Allow your imagination to run riot. Think about what you have always wanted to do but never quite had the freedom to do before now. That is exactly how this book came to be.

## *Are you serious? I'm disabled!*

A severely disabled man named Torab Bezchi applied to my organization in 1991 to be professionally trained as a stress counsellor. His problem was that he was confined to a wheelchair and would remain so for the rest of his life. We trained him and oversaw the adaptation of his office at home to a consulting room for clients. Obviously, because he became easily tired, he could only counsel a small number of clients each week, so his earning capacity was limited. But the quality of his care was exceptional and his practice built up an excellent reputation.

I had the pleasure of meeting his family one evening at the LCI Practitioner of the Year Awards. They told me how tremendously proud he was to be contributing to the family budget and to be doing something beneficial for others. Only a few months ago I phoned him to check on his progress. I was delighted to hear that his voice sounds stronger and more self-assured, his confidence is high and his practice, he tells me, is getting an increasing number of referrals and recommendations from previous clients.

# 5: The peak of recovery

*Time is the great physician.*

Benjamin Disraeli 1804–81

'The peak of recovery? When will I get there?' I used to believe, based upon medical opinion, that three years after stroke, you will be as well as you are ever going to get. Well, it's true that on the third anniversary of my second stroke, I felt almost completely recovered. My only two remaining deficits at that time were that I still needed a Mediterranean-type siesta during the afternoon in order to make it through to the end of the day, and my ability to pronounce words with precision deteriorated rapidly if I became tired or flustered.

Now, as I approach my fourth anniversary of stroke, those deficits remain but I feel healthier and more energized than ever. If I go on getting any better, I shall end up better than I was prior to my illness.

Is that really so surprising? I don't think so. I realized early on that self-help, laughter and faith in my ability to pick myself up from the depths of despair were qualities that would get me through. I have worked hard and sacrificed much to regain my health. I have followed my doctor's advice to the letter and changed my previously enjoyable but unhealthy lifestyle for my existing enjoyable but healthy lifestyle. I have done nothing heroic; I simply refused to give in to a couple of strokes because I love life and had every intention of continuing to do so.

From my stress management days, I knew that the human mind can exercise a lot more power than the body. Many of those clients, before therapy, had somehow managed to convince themselves (or allowed someone else to convince them) that they had a problem, physical or otherwise, for which there

**THE BOTTOM LINE**

Time + the will to get well = maximum recovery.

was little hope of a solution. Sadly, with stroke illness, many people defeat themselves because they are too afraid to even try to get better.

Everything I have done to recover from stroke, without exception, is detailed in this book. Please go ahead and benefit as much as possible from my experience. Go on getting better and better yourself. Better than you have been for years! Who is to say when you will achieve the peak of your recovery? And could it be higher than you ever thought possible?

# 6: Next generation drugs

> *The widespread misconception that 'nothing can be done about stroke' is being swept aside as new prospects for prevention, acute treatment and rehabilitation come to the fore.*
>
> 1998 Scrip Report on Stroke:
> 'Pathways to Future Therapy' by Ruth Kirby

Treatment for stroke is developing all the time. Although stroke remains a huge hurdle for modern medicine, it is now known that brain tissue can be salvaged if blood flow is re-established quickly. As I write, the first transplant of manufactured human brain cells is taking place in Pittsburgh, USA.

## The future is brighter for stroke patients

There is an emerging trend towards specialist stroke units and more positive management, both in prevention and treatment of stroke. Major efforts are

**THE BOTTOM LINE**

Future prospects for stroke patients are encouraging.

under way to educate the public about the warning symptoms of the illness and the emergency nature of stroke. Slogans such as 'time is brain' are even being employed within the medical community to enforce this all-important message.

When stroke interrupts the blood flow to the brain, lack of oxygen kills cells by triggering a cascade of chemical reactions. Several major drug companies around the world are optimistic that they will develop an effective drug to block these toxic chemicals. This will represent a tremendous breakthrough in limiting the extent of brain damage caused by stroke.

---

### Emerging research and new millennium therapies

- Tiny pieces of tissue travelling in the bloodstream can easily get lodged in a small blood vessel. If this occurs in the head it can lead to a stroke. Research in Britain is currently taking place using a special ultrasound technique to try to detect patients who are at high risk of this type of stroke so that preventive measures can be taken early.

- Magnetic Resonance Imaging can now be used to give safe and accurate images of the arteries to the brain. In ongoing clinical trials, clot-busters are injected straight into blood clots through long and thin flexible tubes called catheters. The catheter is inserted into the femoral artery in the groin, then manipulated up into the brain so that the drug can be directed at the clot to dissolve it.

- Intense research internationally is continuing for an effective neuroprotective drug to reduce the extent of brain damage in stroke.

# 7: Courage

*Great emergencies and crises show us how much greater our vital resources are than we had supposed.*

William James 1842–1910

Serious illness subjects us to extreme discomfort, anxiety and frustration. Of patients with the capacity to recover, those patients who recuperate best have one quality in common – courage. This extraordinary quality is the hallmark of both the effective carer and the determined stroke survivor. It is often displayed by ordinary men and women, usually when their lives are turned upside down by some unexpected catastrophe and they are battling against overwhelming odds. Courage is not the exclusive preserve of heroes. The most unlikely people are capable of showing immense courage should they be sufficiently incensed or inspired to care passionately about something or someone.

I did not discover my own courage easily. My commitment to recovery was born of weakness, *vanity* in fact. After my second stroke in hospital, only three days after my first, I found it hard to believe that the semi-dependent babbler I had become was *me*.

I was particularly affronted by the realization that one side of my mouth was a full inch higher than the other. For me, no price was too high, no effort too great, to win back my health. I would have done anything to bring back some semblance of normality to my life. Indeed I did. Prompted by fear of the future, vanity and sheer bloody-mindedness, I blundered persistently onwards to almost total recovery over the next three years.

IN RETROSPECT, I REALIZE NOW THAT I HAD FOUND THE WILL TO GET WELL.

**THE BOTTOM LINE**

# Have you seen this quotation before?
# Let's act on it!

Patients who are highly committed to recovery are consistently better able to withstand setbacks than those to whom existence is simply a burden. The same is true of carers who are motivated and committed to the task in hand. Similarly, those who exercise a degree of control over their reaction to adversity do better than those who feel they are powerless victims of circumstance. This does not mean that we must control all of the events affecting us. As stroke patients and carers that would be impossible, but it does mean that we should exercise control over *how we react.*

Life can seem cruel and unfair at times. Understandably, we wonder why disaster has befallen us. Nevertheless, those individuals who accept the challenge to win back their health or care for a loved one are more likely to succeed than those who see themselves as victims. Patients with a clear sense of direction and purpose in recovery and rehabilitation fare better than those without. Commit your heart and soul to the challenge of making the best possible recovery available to you and **you will succeed.**

# 8: My resolution

My name is: .............................................................................................................

From now on, my purpose in life is: ......................................................................

..............................................................................................................................

Now that I have read this book, *I am going to*: ...................................................

..............................................................................................................................

The help I need most *is*: ........................................................................................

..............................................................................................................................

# 9: My resolution as carer

Now that I have read this book *I am going to*: .................................................

.................................................................................................................

The chapters that mean most to me *are*: .................................................

.................................................................................................................

The personal support I need most *is*: .................................................

.................................................................................................................

The people who will help and support me *are*: .................................................

.................................................................................................................

The professional assistance I need most *is*: .................................................

.................................................................................................................

(Please refer to the pages that follow.)

**THE BOTTOM LINE**

I wish both patient and carer well. I sincerely
hope this book has been helpful.

# Sources of help and support

## *United Kingdom*

**The Stroke Association**
Stroke House, Whitecross Street
London EC1Y 8JJ
Telephone (020) 7490 7999/7566 0300 Fax (020) 7490 2686
*e-mail address: stroke@stroke.org.uk*
*website http://www.stroke.org.uk*

**Chest Heart and Stroke Scotland**
65 North Castle Street
Edinburgh EH2 3LT
Telephone (0131) 225 6963 Fax (0131) 220 6313 Edinburgh
(0141) 633 1666 Fax (0141) 633 5113 Glasgow
(01463) 713 433 Fax (01463) 713 699 Inverness

**Northern Ireland Chest Heart and Stroke Association**
21 Dublin Road
Belfast BT2 7HB
Telephone (028) 9032 0184 Fax (028) 9033 3487 Helpline (0345) 697299
*e-mail address: mail@nichsa.com*
*website http://www.nichsa.com*

**Different Strokes**
Sir Walter Scott House
2 Broadway Market
London E8 4QJ
Telephone (020) 7249 6645 Fax (020) 7249 0881

**Chartered Society of Physiotherapy**
14 Bedford Row
London WC1R 4ED
Telephone (020) 7306 6666 Fax (020) 7306 6611

**RADAR – Royal Association for Disability and Rehabilitation**
12 City Forum
250 City Road
London EC1V 8AF
Telephone (020) 7250 3222 Fax (020) 7250 0212

**Disabled Living Foundation**
380–384 Harrow Road
London W9 2HU
Telephone (020) 7289 6111 Fax (020) 7266 2922

**The Disability Information Trust**
Mary Marlborough Centre
Nuffield Orthopaedic Centre
Headington, Oxford OX3 7LD
Telephone (01865) 227592 Fax (01865) 227596

**Royal College of Speech and Language Therapists**
7 Bath Place
Rivington Street
London EC2A 3DR
Telephone (020) 7613 3855 Fax (020) 7613 3854

**Keep Able**
Fleming Close
Park Close, Park Farm
Wellingborough, Northants NN8 3BR
Telephone (01933) 679426

**Mobility Information Service**
National Mobility Centre
Unit 2a Atcham Estate
Shrewsbury SY4 4UG
Telephone (01743) 761889 Fax (01743) 761149

**Continence Foundation**
2 Doughty Street
London WC1N 2PH
Telephone (020) 7404 6875 Helpline (0191) 213 0050 Fax (020) 404 6876

**Action for Dysphasic Adults**
1 Royal Street
London SE1 7LL
Telephone (020) 7261 9572 Fax (020) 7928 9542

**British Aphasiology Society**
Department of Clinical Communication Studies
City University
Northampton Square
London EC1V 0HB
Telephone (020) 7477 8000 extension 4668

**Age Concern**
1268 London Road
London SW16 4ER
Telephone (020) 8679 8000 National Information Hotline 0800 009966

**British Association for Counselling**
1 Regent Place
Rugby
Warwickshire CV21 2PJ
Telephone (01788) 578328

**Carers' National Association**
20–25 Glasshouse Yard
London EC1 4JS
Telephone (020) 7490 8818

**La' Viva Weighted Body Garments**
The Yewberry
Yewberry Lane, Newport
South Wales NP9 6WL
Telephone (01633) 822012

**Crossroads – Association of Care Attendant Schemes Ltd**
10 Regent Place
Rugby
Warwickshire CV21 2PN
Telephone (01788) 573653 Fax (01788) 565498

**Department of Social Security Disability Unit**
The Adelphi
1–11 John Adam Street
London WC2N 6HT
Telephone (020) 7712 2062 Fax (020) 7712 2075

**Disability Alliance**
1st Floor East, Universal House
88–94 Wentworth Street
London E1 7SA
Telephone (020) 7247 8763

**Disabled Drivers' Association**
Ashwellthorpe
Norwich NR16 1EX
Telephone (01508) 489449 Fax (01508) 488173

**John Grooms Association for Disabled People**
10 Gloucester Drive
Finsbury Park
London N4 2LP
Telephone (020) 8802 7272 Fax (020) 8809 1754

**Mavis – Mobility Advice and Vehicle Information Service**
Crowthorne
Berkshire RG45 6AU
Telephone (01344) 770456 Fax (01344) 770692

**Motability**
2nd Floor, Gate House
Harlow
Essex CM20 1HR
Telephone (01279) 635999 Fax (01279) 635677 Customer Services Helpline
    (01279) 635666

**College of Occupational Therapists**
6–8 Marshalsea Road
London SE1 1HL
Telephone (020) 7357 6480

**National Association of Citizens' Advice Bureaux**
115–123 Pentonville Road
London N1 9LZ
Telephone (020) 7833 2181 Fax (020) 7833 4371

**Managing Migraine**
Freepost
PO Box 21
Godalming
Surrey GU7 2BR

## *Republic of Ireland*

**The Volunteer Stroke Scheme**
249 Crumlin Road
Dublin 12
Telephone (01) 455 9036/455 7455 Fax (01) 455 7013

**NRB – National Rehabilitation Board**
Upper Mallow Street
Limerick
Telephone (061) 319779/314270 Fax (061) 412977

**NRH – National Rehabilitation Hospital**
Speech and Language Therapy Department
Rochestown Avenue
Dun Laoghaire, Co. Dublin
Telephone (01) 285 4777 Fax (01) 285 1053

**IASLT – Irish Association of Speech and Language Therapists**
4 Argus House, Greenmount Office Park
Harolds Cross Road, Dublin 6
Telephone (01) 473 0398

**Irish Wheelchair Association**
Arus Churchlain, Black Heath Drive
Dublin 3
Telephone (01) 833 3884

## Australia

**National Stroke Foundation**
Level 11, 167 Queen Street
Melbourne, Victoria 3000
Telephone (61) 3 9670 1000 Fax (61) 3 9670 9300
*e-mail address: jim@natstroke.asn.au*
*website http://www.natstroke.asn.au*

**Australian Brain Foundation**
Suite 21, Regent House,
Alexander Street, Crow's Nest, NSW 2065
Telephone 9437 5967 Fax 9437 5978

**Stroke Association of Victoria**
721 Barkley Street
Ballarat, VIC 3350
Telephone (053) 31 3969

**Carers Association of NSW**
Level 5, 93 York Street
Sydney, NSW 2000
Telephone 9299 1499 Fax 9299 1022

**Carers Association of Western Australia**
Selby Ctr., 2 Selby Street
Shenton Park, WA 6008
Telephone (09) 380 4900 Fax (09) 382 0817

**Department of Rehabilitation Medicine**
L2 QE 11 Rehabilitation Centre
RPAH, 59 Missenden Road
Camperdown, NSW 2050
Telephone 9515 9815 Fax 9515 9750

**Hunter Outreach Centre**
Charlestown Multipurpose Centre
17 James Street
Charlestown 2290
Telephone (049) 439 786

**Stroke Association of Western Australia**
P.O. Box 308
Bentley 6102
Telephone (09) 451 8071

**Support, Self-Help and Social Activities for Stroke People in Queensland**
P.O. Box 426
Morningside, QLD 4170
Telephone (07) 3399 9461

**Neurological Resource Centre**
23a King William Road
Unley, SA 5061
Telephone (08) 357 8919

**Stroke Club of Tasmania**
10 Maritana Place
Claremont, TAS 7011
Telephone (002) 492 033 (Mrs Val Mason)

## New Zealand

**Stroke Foundation of New Zealand Inc.**
National Office, Level 1, Federation House
95–99 Molesworth Street
P.O. Box 12482
Wellington
Telephone (04) 472 8099 Fax (04) 472 7019 Freephone 0800 787653
*e-mail address: strokenz@voyager.co.nz*

**Stroke Foundation of New Zealand Inc.**
177 Victoria Road
St Kilda, Dunedin
Telephone (03) 455 8613

**Stroke Foundation of New Zealand Inc.**
P.O. Box 31237
Milford Auckland
Telephone (09) 486 0899

**Stroke Foundation of New Zealand Inc. Southern Region**
314 Worcester Street
Christchurch
Telephone (03) 377 1294

**Stroke Foundation of New Zealand Inc.**
104 Dee Street
Christchurch Invercargill
Telephone (03) 214 5439

**Stroke Foundation of New Zealand Inc. Otago Sub-Region**
4 Dovedale Place,
Hamilton
Telephone (07) 847 4106

## *United States of America*

**Stroke Connection**
American Heart Association
7272 Greenville Avenue
Dallas, Texas 75231
Telephone (800) 553 6321 and (214) 373 6300 Fax (214) 696 5211
*e-mail address: strokeconnection@heart.org*
*website http://www.amhrt.org/stroke/recovery*

**The National Stroke Association**
96 Inverness Drive East, Suite 1
Englewood, Colorado, 80112
Telephone (303) 649 9299 Fax (303) 649 1328

**National Aphasia Association**
156 Fifth Avenue, Suite 707
New York 10010
Telephone (800) 922 4622

**The National Rehabilitation Hospital**
102 Irving Street NW
Washington DC. 20010
Telephone (202) 877 1000 Fax (202) 726 8512

**National Organisation on Disability**
910 16th Street NW, Suite 600
Washington DC. 20006
Telephone (202) 293 5960 and (800) 248 2253

**National Rehabilitation Information Center**
8455 Colesville Road, Suite 935
Silver Springs, MD 20910
Telephone (301) 588 9284 and (800) 346 2742

**The National Eastern Seal Society**
70 East Lake Street
Chicago, Illinois 60601
Telephone (312) 726 6200 Fax (312) 726 1494

**American Occupational Therapy Association**
1383 Piccard Drive
P.O. Box 1725, Rockville MD 20849
Telephone (301) 948 9626

**American Physical Therapy Association**
1111 North Fairfax Street
Alexandria, VA 22314
Telephone (703) 684 2782

**American Speech-Language-Hearing Association**
10801 Rockville Pike
Rockville MD 20852
Telephone (800) 638 8255

**The National Stroke and Quality of Life Medical Institute**
630 West 168th Street
New York, 10032
Telephone (914) 779 4877 Fax (718) 802 0180

**Carbrillo College Stroke Center**
501 Upper Park Road
Santa Cruz, California 95065
Telephone (408) 425 0622 Fax (408) 425 0223

**Palm Springs Stroke Activity Center**
2800 East Alego Road
Palm Springs, California 92268
Telephone (619) 323 7676 Fax (619) 325 8026

**The United Stroke Program Inc.**
13530 Aviation Boulevard
Hawthorne, CA 90250
Telephone (213) 643 5195

**American Rehabilitation Association**
P.O. Box 17675
Washington DC. 20006
Telephone (202) 737 8300

**Information Center for Individuals with Disabilities**
20 Park plaza, Room 330
Boston MA 02116
Telephone (800) 462 5015

**National Association of Area Agencies on Ageing**
1112 16th Street NW, Suite 100
Washington DC. 20036
Telephone (202) 296 8130 and (800) 677 1116

**National Council on the Ageing**
409 3rd Street SW, 2nd floor
Washington DC. 20024
Telephone (202) 479 1200 and (800) 424 9046

## *Canada*

**Heart and Stroke Foundation of Canada**
222 Queen Street, Suite 1402
Ottawa, Ontario K1P 5V9
Telephone (613) 569 4361 Fax (613) 569 3278

**Canadian Stroke Recovery Association**
170 The Donway West, Suite 122
Don Mills, Ontario M3C 2G3
Telephone (416) 446 1580

**Stroke Association of British Columbia**
1645 West 10th Avenue
Vancouver BC V6J 2A2
Telephone (604) 734 3616

**SAM – Stroke Association of Manitoba Inc.**
1–3 Vaughan Street
Manitoba R3B 3J9
Telephone (204) 942 2880

**The Heart and Stroke Foundation of Ontario**
474 Mount Pleasant Road, 4th floor
Toronto M45 2L9
Telephone (416) 489 7100 and (800) 360 1557

**The Heart and Stroke Foundation of Quebec**
465 Rene Levesque Boulevard, 3rd Floor
Montreal H3Z 1A8
Telephone (514) 871 1551 Fax (514) 871 1464

**The Aphasia Centre**
53 The Links Road
North York, Ontario M2P 1T7
Telephone (416) 226 3636 Fax (416) 226 3706

# South Africa

**Stroke Aid/*Beroete Hulp***
PO Box 51283, Raedene 2124, Johannesburg
Telephone (011) 788 2404 Mrs Tommy Reinecke (011) 882 1612
    Mrs Shirley Abrams (011) 442 7546 Mrs Adrienne White

**Stroke Aid/*Beroete Hulp***
1880 Butshingi Street
Dube Village
Soweto, 1800
Telephone (011) 982 2720 Mrs Mavis Tshabalala

**Association for the Physically Disabled (Western Cape)**
P.O. Box/Postbus 1375
Cape Town/Kaapstad 8000
Telephone (021) 685 4153

**Cape Peninsular Organisation**
Private Bag 7
Newlands, 7725
Telephone (021) 686 7830

**Highway Aged/Stroke Club**
42 Kings Road
Pinetown, 3600, Durban
Telephone (031) 701 5571

**TAFTA – The Association for the Aged**
P.O. Box/Postbus 2983
Durban, 4000
Telephone (031) 465 1860

# Index